Hèla Ben Jmaà
Abir Bouassida
Tarak Ben Jmaà

Cardio-pericardial hydatid cysts

Hèla Ben Jmaà
Abir Bouassida
Tarak Ben Jmaà

Cardio-pericardial hydatid cysts

Cardiac hydatid cysts

ScienciaScripts

Imprint

Any brand names and product names mentioned in this book are subject to trademark, brand or patent protection and are trademarks or registered trademarks of their respective holders. The use of brand names, product names, common names, trade names, product descriptions etc. even without a particular marking in this work is in no way to be construed to mean that such names may be regarded as unrestricted in respect of trademark and brand protection legislation and could thus be used by anyone.

Cover image: www.ingimage.com

This book is a translation from the original published under ISBN 978-620-6-71652-5.

Publisher:
Sciencia Scripts
is a trademark of
Dodo Books Indian Ocean Ltd. and OmniScriptum S.R.L publishing group

120 High Road, East Finchley, London, N2 9ED, United Kingdom
Str. Armeneasca 28/1, office 1, Chisinau MD-2012, Republic of Moldova, Europe
Printed at: see last page
ISBN: 978-620-7-86240-5

Table of contents

I- Introduction :

Hydatid disease or hydatidosis is a cosmopolitan parasitic infection caused by the development in humans of the larval form of a dog taenia: *Echinococcus granulosus* (1).

Man is an accidental host, taking the place of the herbivore.

The geographical distribution of this pathology is directly linked to human-dog-sheep contact.

It is endemic in certain areas of the world, such as the Mediterranean basin. It is a real public health problem in Tunisia. (2) (3).

It can affect all organs. Hepatic localization is the most frequent, followed by pulmonary localization.

Cardio-pericardial hydatidosis is much rarer, accounting for 0.5% to 2% of all visceral localizations. (4).

Hydatidosis can develop in any tunica of the heart.

Hydatid cysts of the heart are a serious condition, with local and general complications that can be life-threatening.

The clinical presentation, treatment and prognosis of cardiac hydatidosis depend mainly on the tunica involved and the rate of development of the parasitic collection.

II- Parasitological review :

1. The pathogen (5) :

The taenia Echinococcus Granulosus is a cestode of the plathelminth family. It comes in three evolutionary forms:

-       The adult form: lives attached between the villi of the small intestine of the definitive host.

-       The ovular or egg form: this is the externalized form of the parasite, which survives in the external environment and contaminates the intermediate host and man.

-       The hydatid larva: This is a more or less spherical, fluid-filled vesicle that develops in the infested organ of the intermediate host or human.

2. The parasite cycle (5) (6) :

The parasite cycle is mainly domestic, involving two hosts:

-       A definitive host represented essentially by the dog.

-       An intermediate host, represented by sheep, cattle, goats and pigs.

The embryonated eggs, eliminated into the environment with the dog's feces, are ingested by the intermediate host.

In the latter's small intestine, under the action of digestive juices, the embryo attaches itself to the intestinal wall, which it crosses to enter the portal system. It is then carried by the portal current to the liver, where it may pass through the supra-hepatic veins to reach the lungs.

More rarely, it may localize to any of the body's viscera via the general circulation, such as the heart, spleen, bone...

Echinococcus granulosus larvae escape the hepatic filter and enter the left heart chambers, then the right atrium and left heart via the pulmonary circulation or a permeable foramen ovale. (7).

From the left ventricle, the larvae are expelled into the large circulation and, via the coronary arteries, the parasite invades the myocardium. (8).

Once inside the viscera, the embryo transforms into a hydatid larva (Figure 1).

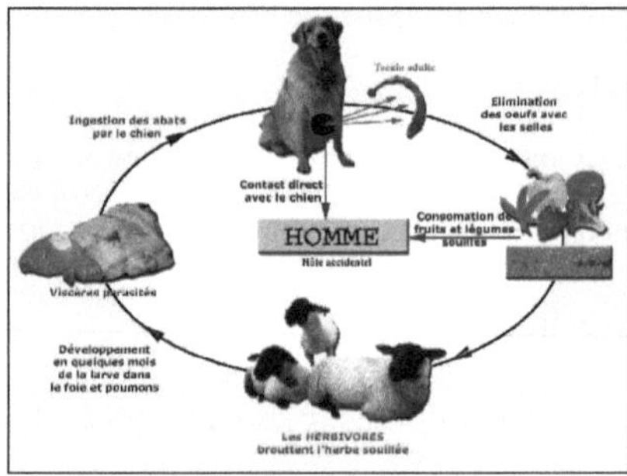

Figure 1: Parasitic cycle of Echinococcus Granulosus (9).

3. Methods of contamination (6):

The definitive host becomes infected by devouring the infested viscera of the intermediate host.

The intermediate host becomes infected by ingesting pasture soiled with eggs. Man is an accidental host, taking the sheep's place. Contamination occurs via the digestive tract, in two ways:

- Direct contamination through close contact with parasitized dogs.
- Indirect contamination through ingestion of contaminated food.

By becoming infected, man constitutes a parasitic dead end in the hydatid cyst cycle.

III- Historical background (10) (11) (12):

- Although hydatid disease has been known since the time of Hippocrates, the first description of cardiac hydatidosis was in 1846 by Griesinger (10).

- Marten and De Crespign first attempted surgical treatment in 1921 (11).

- Long successfully performed the first surgical resection without extracorporeal circulation in 1932 (12).

- In 1961, extracorporeal circulation was first used for surgery on cardiac hydatidosis.

IV- Epidemiology:

1. General frequency :

Hydatidosis is a cosmopolitan parasitosis that occurs worldwide (13) (14). Because of its mode of transmission, it is endemic mainly in sheep-breeding countries (15) (16).

It is found mainly in North Africa, in the Maghreb countries and in East Africa, where prevalence is the highest in the world (5) (17).

In Tunisia, hydatidosis is endemic and constitutes a real public health problem (2). The north-western and central-western regions of the country are the most affected (18).

Hepatic localization is by far the most frequent, followed by pulmonary localization. Other localizations are much rarer.

Cardiac localization is estimated at 0.5 to 2% of all hydatid localizations (19) (13) (1).

Its rarity can be explained by the need to cross the hepatic and pulmonary barriers, and by the cardiac contractions that constitute a natural resistance to cyst viability (13).

Cardiac involvement is isolated in 50% of cases, and is not associated with other hepatic, pulmonary or other localizations. It is associated with other sites in 50% of cases (7).

The frequency of the most frequent hydatid localizations is shown in Table I :

Table n° I: Frequency of different hydatidosis localizations (9).

Cyst site	Frequency of location (%)

Liver	70 à 75
Lung	25
Pleura and peritoneum	4 à 7
Kidney	2 à 5
Rate	2 à 5
Brain	1 à 5
Bones	1 à 3
Heart	*0.5 à 2*

2. Frequency by location :

2. 1 The right atrium :

The right atrium is involved in 3 to 4% of cases (7) .

2. 2. The atrial septum:

The atrial septum is affected in 2% of cases (20). The first case described in the literature dates back to 1964 (21). Since then, several other cases have been reported (22) (23).

2. 3 The right ventricle :

The right ventricle is affected in 10-15% of cases (7) (24).

The cyst may be intra-cavitary or intra-parietal. Parietal cysts are subendocardial in 2/3 of right ventricular cysts, due to the thinness of the muscular wall and the low pressure regime in the right cavities, explaining the possibility of intracavitary rupture in 88% of cases. (7).

The cyst may be flush with both the endocardium and epicardium, since the thickness of the right ventricular wall is less than that of the left.

2. 4 The left atrium :

The left atrium is generally involved in 5 to 8% of cases (25).

2.5 The interventricular septum :

Hydatid localization in the interventricular septum is found in 5 to 9% of cases of cardiac hydatidosis (26) (27).

2. 6 The left ventricle :

The most frequent site of cardiac echinococcosis is the left ventricle, due to its greater vascularity and thickness (28) (1). It accounts for 60% of all cardiac localizations. The apex region is the most affected (29).

The cyst may be intracavitary or located in the thickness of the ventricular wall.

In the thickness of the myocardium, it can be :

-   Subepicardial: in 75% of left ventricular cysts, explaining the possibility of intrapericardial rupture (30).
-   Sub-endocardial: much less frequent than sub-epicardial cysts. This location entails a risk of rupture in the left ventricle in 37% of cases (30).

2. 7 The pericardium :

The pericardium is affected in 8% of cases (26).

Isolated pericardial localization without associated cardiac involvement is extremely rare. (4) (8).

Elkarimia S et al (4) described a case of pericardial hydatid cyst revealed by tamponade without associated cardiac localization in a 60-year-old patient.

The frequency of the various cardiac locations of hydatid cysts is shown in Table II :

Table II: Frequency of different cardiac localizations of hydatid cysts (27).

Location	Frequency (%)
Left ventricle	60
Right ventricle	10 à 15
Left auricle	5 à 8
Right auricle	3 à 4
Interventricular septum	5 à 9
Inter-auricular septum	2
Pericardium	8

2. 8. valve location :

Valvular involvement is exceptional.

Sensoz Y et al (31) described a case of a hydatid cyst of the right ventricle invading the posterior leaflet of the tricuspid valve, whose surgical resection required resection of the tricuspid valve and its replacement by a bioprosthesis.

Aksakal E et al (32) reported the first case of a hydatid cyst invading the posterior leaflet of the mitral valve, measuring 2 cm in diameter, in a 60-

year-old woman. The cyst was complicated by mitral narrowing and congestive heart failure.

2. 9. multiple cardiac locations :

The simultaneous presence of several hydatid cysts in the heart is not uncommon. Thameur H et al (33) in a series of 45 cases, reported multiple cardiac hydatid localizations in 12 cases (27%).

2. 10. Association with other extra-cardiac hydatid localizations :

Multi-visceral echinococcosis with cardiac involvement is not exceptional (34). It can reach 40% in some series (35) (36).

3. Terrain :

3. 1 Age :

In most series, the average age of patients is between 30 and 40 years (37). This pathology is rare in the paediatric population (38).

3. 2. gender :

Some publications point to a predominance of the male sex (39) .

V- Pathophysiology of cardiac hydatidosis (40):

Once the hexacanth embryo has been digested, it pierces the intestinal wall with its 6 hooks and enters the portal or lymphatic circulation.

In most cases, the embryo is arrested in the liver, but if not, it passes through or around it, and may be blocked in the pulmonary filter.

After crossing the liver, the embryo reaches the right heart chambers via the suprahepatic veins and inferior vena cava, and can then penetrate the right heart muscle or reach the left heart via the pulmonary circulation or the patent foramen ovale.

After passing through the pulmonary filter, the parasite is routed via the pulmonary veins to the left atrium and left ventricle, where it can then enter the coronary network.

The parasite can also pass through the thoracic duct, shunting the hepatic filter. The thoracic duct empties into the superior vena cava, enabling the parasite to reach the right heart chambers.

<h2 style="text-align:center">VI- Clinical study :</h2>

1. Circumstances of discovery :

The cardiac hydatid cyst is characterized by a low-noise evolution and a long clinical latency due to its slow growth.

There is no characteristic clinical picture, and symptomatology varies according to the size of the cyst, its stage of evolution, its location in relation to the valvular orifices and conduction tissue, and its location in the right or left heart (28).

Thus, hydatid cysts may be compressive, suggesting a valvular obstruction, or an ischemic pathology.

Functional signs are not specific to hydatid cysts of the heart. They are highly variable, depending on the cardiac location, size and number of cysts, and often reflect a complication.

- Dyspnea: its intensity varies from moderate dyspnea to acute respiratory distress. It is mainly seen in cases of tamponade complicating the rupture of a pericardial hydatid cyst (19)or hydatid pulmonary embolism (41) (42).

- Chest pain: this is often precordialgia, which seems to reflect irritation of the pericardium, congestive heart failure, or ischemia of the pericardial zone.

Anginal pain may also be present, reflecting myocardial ischemia caused by compression of the coronary arteries (41) (43).

Pain may also be associated with pericarditis (44).

- Palpitations: These reflect the occurrence of cardiac rhythm disturbances resulting from the cyst's compression of conduction tissue and

the surrounding myocardium (45) (46). They occur in around 22% of cases
(47).

- Syncope: Syncope may be inaugural, pointing to conduction pathway
damage associated with interventricular septal localization (48) or a severe
ventricular rhythm disorder.

Obstruction of the VD ejection pathways can lead to syncope.

- Cough: a frequent sign of hydatid pulmonary embolism secondary to
rupture of a right heart hydatid cyst in the pulmonary artery (28) (42) (49).
It is a persistent, hacking cough, usually dry.

- Hemoptysis: the most important sign of hydatid pulmonary
embolism (50) (49) (42).

- Allergic manifestations: These are related to hyper-sensitivity to
hydatid antigens, occurring following cyst rupture. Their severity varies
from simple urticaria to fatal anaphylactic shock (51).

- Signs associated with systemic hydatid embolism: Systemic
embolism may be indicative of cardiac hydatid localization.

- General signs: Fever is a non-specific sign that may be secondary to
infection of the cyst contents. It may also be associated with anaphylactic
reactions (52).

- Incidental finding: Hydatid cysts of the heart are characterized by
their long clinical latency, which may persist for several years. This latency
is more frequent in cases of left ventricular localization, as cysts grow in
thick muscle (53).

The diagnosis is made by chance, during a systematic paraclinical
examination, or during the extension of a pulmonary or hepatic hydatidosis.

2. Physical examination :

Physical examination is of little value in the diagnosis of cardiac hydatidosis.

Physical signs are rarely found and are not specific.

These may include :

- A muffling of heart sounds.
- The discovery of a systolic or diastolic murmur on auscultation due to valve damage (44).
- Physical examination is of little value in the diagnosis of cardiac hydatidosis.
- Physical signs are rarely found and are not specific.

These may include :

- A muffling of heart sounds.
- The discovery of a systolic or diastolic murmur on auscultation due to valve damage (44).

VII- Paraclinical examinations :

Clinical diagnosis of uncomplicated hydatid cysts of the heart is difficult due to the lack of specificity of functional signs (45).

Paraclinical examinations enable the diagnosis to be made in 80% of cases preoperatively (54).

1. Chest X-ray:

Chest X-rays may show no significant abnormalities, in which case the cyst may be small or develop exclusively within the cavity. (19).

The frontal chest X-ray may show a mediastinal syndrome with :

-       Cardiomegaly.

-       A round or oval opacity, watery in tone, homogeneous, deforming the contours of the heart, most often the left lower arch (figure no. 2).

-       Calcifications may be present, outlining the opacity.

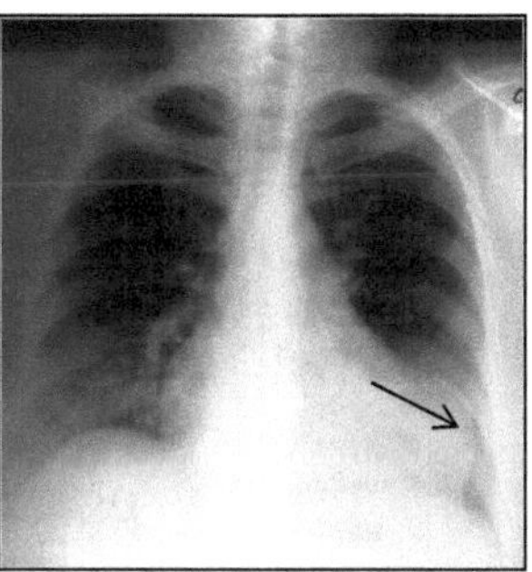

Figure 2: Front thoracic X-ray showing a protrusion of the left inferior arch of the heart in connection with a hydatid cyst of the left ventricle (arrow) (48).

They are likely to be associated with pulmonary hydatid cysts, which is why it is advisable to look for them on a thoracic radiograph with front and side views. They appear as round or oval opacities, single or multiple, fluid in tone, homogeneous or heterogeneous, depending on the stage of hydatid cyst evolution. (55).

Chest X-rays may also show signs of pulmonary overload or edema.

2. Electrocardiogram :

The electrical response to hydatid cysts of the heart varies according to the location of the cyst, its stage of development, and any complications it may cause.

A normal recording may be seen. ECG abnormalities are observed in 40% of cases. These abnormalities may be :

2. 1 Rhythm disorders (56) :

The most frequently observed rhythm disorders are :

- Sinus tachycardia.
- Supraventricular tachycardia.
- Atrial or ventricular extrasystoles.
- Atrial fibrillation.

2. 2. Repolarization disorders (44):

Depending on the location of the cyst and its impact, repolarization disorders may be :

- Of ischemic origin when there is compression of a coronary vessel: this may involve T-wave inversion, or more rarely ST-segment modification in territories dependent on the location of the cyst (figure no. 3).
- Due to intrapericardial rupture: changes in PQ and ST segments.

-       Either non-specific, like inverted T waves, of stable appearance with no evolutionary character, and involving the territory occupied by the cyst.

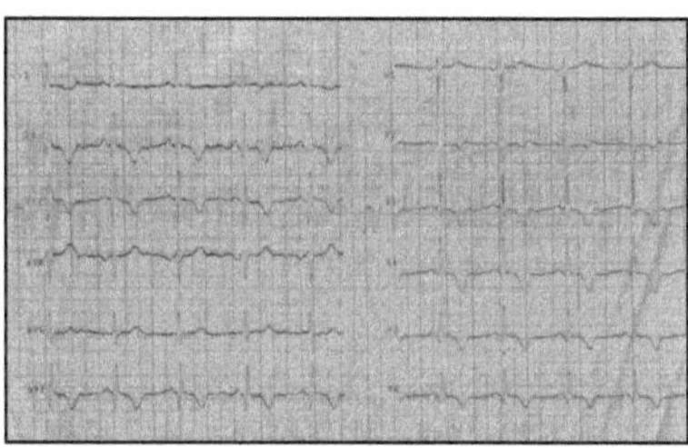

Figure 3: ECG showing T-wave inversion inferiorly and apico-laterally in a patient with a left ventricular hydatid cyst revealed by an inaugural coronary syndrome (44) .

2. 3 Conduction disorders :
They are often associated with lesions of the interventricular septum.

3. Doppler echocardiography :

It is the examination of choice for the diagnosis of hydatid cysts. It should be carried out systematically in the case of visceral echinococcosis, to check for cardiac localization (4).

It enables a positive diagnosis to be made, the size and appearance of the cyst to be determined, and the relationship with adjacent anatomical structures and hemodynamic repercussions to be accurately established, in order to guide therapeutic management (57).

3. 1. Positive diagnosis :

The cyst appears as a single or multiple mass, with a liquid echo-structure or containing daughter vesicles, rounded or oval, with or without a thick shell, depending on the stage of hydatid cyst evolution (58).

The presence of a proligeral membrane with wall detachment and splitting is pathognomonic of hydatidosis (59).

3.2 Impact on adjacent structures:

Doppler ultrasonography can reveal :

- Compression of adjacent heart chambers.
- Compression of the trunk of the pulmonary artery or its branches, hence the importance of Doppler, which can detect a pressure gradient anomaly at this level (60).
- Coronary artery backflow (44).

3.3 Looking for complications :

It can also be used to detect complications such as cracking or rupture, and to study the impact on cardiac function. (58).

- Infected cyst: echo-structured mass of impure tissue or fluid (61).
- Cyst with heterogeneous contents: by rupture of the cyst and emptying of its contents (62) .

3. 4 Specific aspects according to cystic location :

- ***Right atrium:*** Hydatid cysts in the right atrium can obstruct venous return or atrial emptying. Their evolution can be complicated by pulmonary embolisms.

- ***Left atrium:*** Cysts developing in the left atrium are sometimes difficult to differentiate from tumors, especially myxoma, or from intracavitary thrombi, of which the OG is the preferred site.

- ***The atrial septum:*** Hydatid cysts of the AIS often develop in one of the two atria. They may be accompanied by atrial septal defects, either inaugurally or after surgical cure.

- **_Right ventricle:_** The hydatid cyst at this level may be intra-cavitary or intra-parietal.

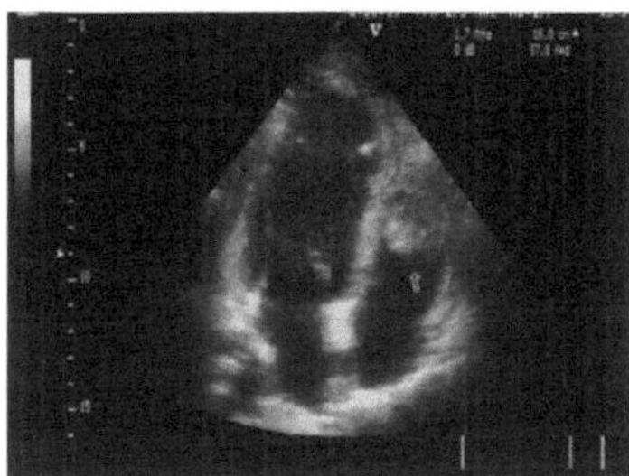

Figure 4: Sonographic appearance of a non-homogeneous cystic mass in the right ventricular cavity (31).

- **_Left ventricle: Most often,_** this is a single cyst that develops intramyocardially, at the expense of the free wall of the ventricle (figure 5).

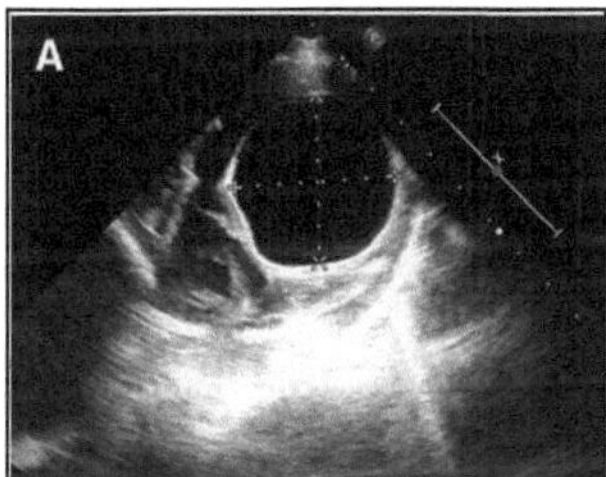

Figure 5: Sonographic appearance of a large hypoechoic cyst in the left ventricular wall (35).

- **_The interventricular septum:_** the septal cyst protrudes into a ventricular cavity (figure 6).

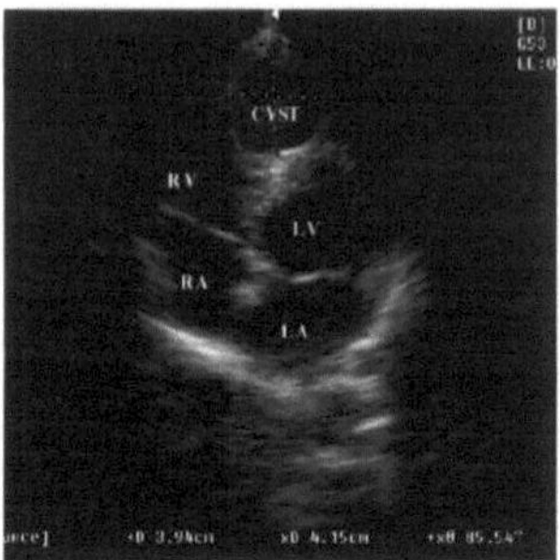

Figure 6: Trans-thoracic ultrasound showing a rounded cystic formation in the interventricular septum (63).

- ***The pericardium:*** Pericardial hydatidosis can take the form of a thin-walled, anechoic formation with pericardial effusion or multi-vesicular appearance, which are highly suggestive of hydatid origin (4) (figure 7).

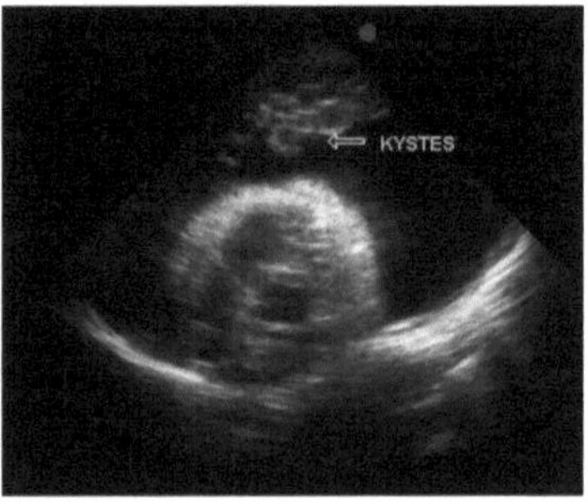

Figure 7: Large pericardial effusion with grape-like cystic formations revealing intrapericardial hydatidosis (4).

3.5 Limitations of echocardiography :

ETT has technical limitations related to imperfect conditions (obesity, poor echogenicity), or due to the remoteness of certain structures (inter-ventricular septum, left atrium) (64).

The sensitivity of TTE is also reduced in the case of masses less than 1 cm in diameter, and in the analysis of complicated cyst contents including membrane remnants and thrombotic material. In these cases, diagnosis is difficult on TTE, and the differential diagnosis with other cardiac tumours is sometimes only anatomical (65) .

4. Computed tomography :

In addition to making a positive diagnosis, the main benefit of CT scanning is that it can be used to assess extension to adjacent structures through thoracoabdominal acquisition, in search of multi-visceral localization (66).

The cyst takes on the appearance of a fluid formation in the cardiac muscle and inside the cavities, showing no change in density after injection of the contrast medium (figure 8). Well-visualized parietal calcifications are inconstant but suggestive (58).

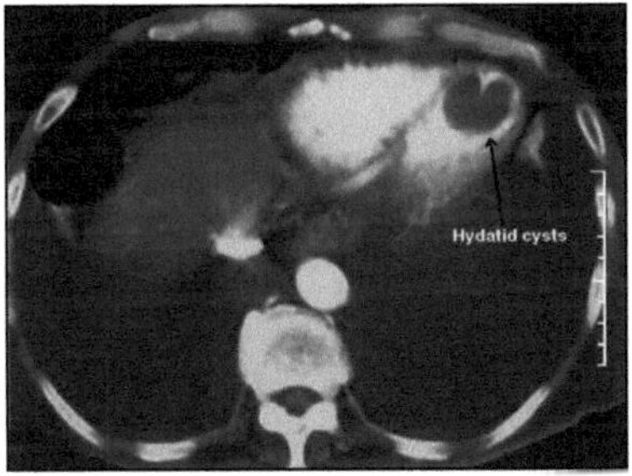

Figure 8: Axial CT scan showing a homogeneous hypodense structure with regular contours that does not enhance with arterial time, located at the apex of the left ventricle (67).

However, artefacts induced by cardiac movements are the main limitation for the CT study of cardiac hydatid cysts.

CT is less effective than echocardiography in pinpointing the location of cardiac hydatid cysts (41) (68). For Ben Hamda et al (47), it provides no additional information compared with echocardiography.

5. MRI (69) (70) :

Thanks to better spatial resolution and the possibility of performing a multi-planar study, MRI is the method of choice for exploring cardiac hydatidosis (58). It has good sensitivity and enables positive diagnosis of small cystic formations (71).

This non-irradiating examination enables a positive diagnosis to be made, thanks to better contrast resolution, and offers the possibility of cross-sectioning in the different planes of space, allowing the cyst site to be better approached. (58).

It can be used to assess mediastinal extension and to search for other liver, spleen and kidney sites.

Typically, the hydatid cyst takes the form of a rounded or oval lesion, hypointense in T1 and hyperintense in T2, with a peripheral contour hypointense in T2 corresponding to the pericyst (figure 9).

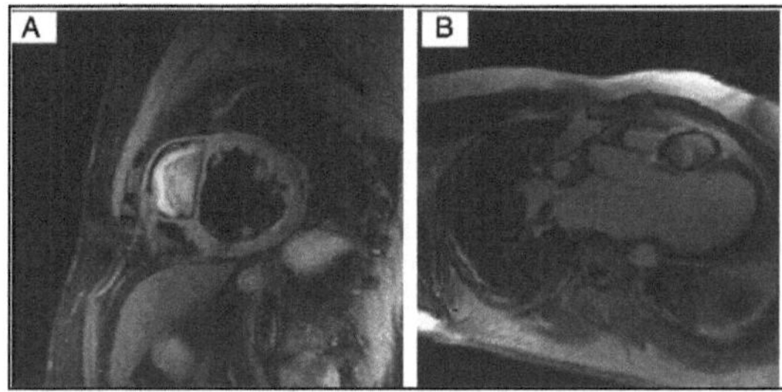

Figure 9: T2 appearance of cyst: hyperintense signal from cyst contents with hypointense signal from pericyst (70).

The acquisition of sections in different planes, with cardiac synchronization, enables the seat diagnosis to be made with certainty.

The study of the impact of cystic masses on cardiac function is made possible by the use of cine-MRI (66).

6. Cardiac catheterization and coronary angiography:

It is not routinely indicated, especially if the hydatid cyst is asymptomatic or uncomplicated.

Coronary angiography enables a detailed study of the coronary arteries and their relationship to the mass, and is necessary in the event of angina manifestations in the patient (33).

Coronary anomalies may be stretch, compression or deviation of a coronary branch, which is the most frequent anomaly (72).

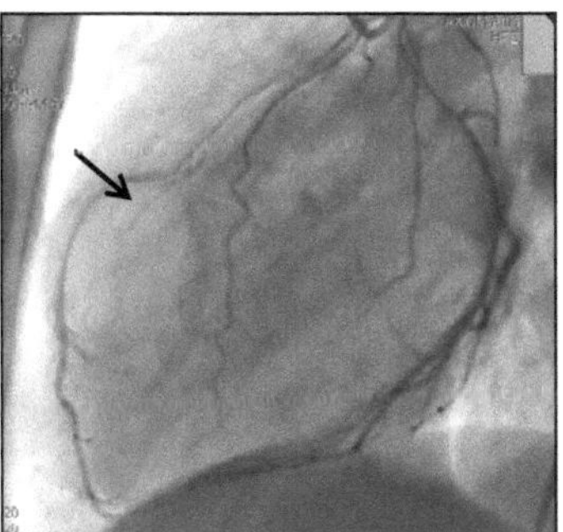

Figure 10: Compression of the distal IVA by a hydatid cyst (arrow) (73).

VIII- Biology :

1. Non-specific examinations :

- **Hyper-eosinophilia:** Inconsistent, found in 23% of cases. It is moderate except in cases of invasion, fissuring or rupture, or during the growth phase of the cyst (74).

- **Increase in total Ig E:** Cestodes cause an increase in serum Ig E levels.

- **Biological assessment of the impact and extension to other organs: The following** may be found:

- Biological inflammatory syndrome (hyperleukocytosis, increased SV).

- Increased cardiac enzymes in cases of myocardial damage.

- Impaired liver function in cases of hepatic localization.

2. Specific examinations :

They are based on immunological diagnosis (75).

- **Specific Ig E assay:** Specific Ig E is a sign of parasitic infection. They are involved in allergic reactions through stimulation of basophil polynuclear cells (76).

Their rate correlates with the progressive stage of the disease (77).

Their levels decrease rapidly after treatment, so they have a role to play in subsequent follow-up and detection of possible recurrences.

- **Serological reactions or serodiagnosis:** Hydatid serology is always required for both diagnostic and post-therapeutic purposes, in order to assess the efficacy of treatment. (75).

ELISA and indirect immunofluorescence are the most sensitive tests. Immunoelectrophoresis is the most specific test (7).

If this test is positive with a significant rate, the diagnosis can be retained. However, if the test is negative, the diagnosis of hydatidosis cannot be formally excluded. Indeed, in some cases, the reaction is falsely negative if the cyst is calcified, or if it is small in size (75).

Rare false-positive reactions may occur in cases of other helminthiases, neoplastic pathology or immune disorders (74).

Serological monitoring of patients enables us to monitor treatment efficacy. After surgical resection, serological negativation is observed within variable timeframes. Re-ascension of antibody levels suggests a risk of recurrence or reinfestation (75).

IX- Histological study :

1. The adult form:

The adult form of the taenia is formed by 3 portions which are the head, the neck, and the body:

- The head, or scolex, consists of 4 rounded suckers and a protruding rostrum armed with a double ring of hooks. The suckers and hooks ensure the parasite's adhesion to the host's intestinal wall. It takes the form of a worm, 2 to 7 mm long, living in a saprophytic state, attached between the villi of the dog's small intestine (figure 11).

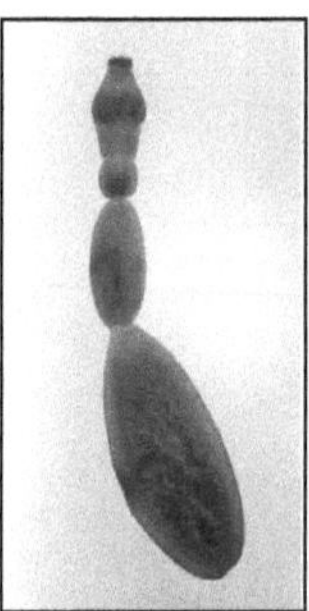

Figure 11: Microscopic appearance of adult Echinococcus Granulosus (78).

- The neck and body of the worm: the body is made up of 3 to 5 rings. When mature, it detaches from the rest of the parasite and is expelled in the stool, releasing the eggs.

2. The oval or egg shape:

The last ring detaches and is evacuated with droppings, releasing the eggs into the surrounding environment.

These eggs or embryophores, measuring 35 to 45μm, contain a hexacanth embryo with 6 hooks.

3. The larval form or hydatid cyst (78) (79):

Its size varies widely, from a few centimetres to over 20 cm in diameter in humans.

From outside to inside, the larval form is made up of :

- Adventitia: formed by parenchyma and the host's inflammatory reaction. It results from compression of the hydatid cyst. The adventitia forms a cleavage zone between the hydatid and the viscera.
- The membrane or anhistatic cuticle: this is the outer wall of the cyst, 1 or 2 mm thick, pearly white and acellular. It has a certain elasticity that allows the cyst to grow.
- The proligeral or germinal membrane: this is the inner wall of the cyst, very thin (20 μm thick), with a syncitial cell layer.
- Proligeral vesicles: 300 to 800 μm in size, they result from the vesiculation of the proligeral membrane on its inner surface.
- They have no cuticular wall and remain attached to the proligera of the mother vesicle by a syncitial pedicle.
- Endogenous daughter vesicles: these result from the vesiculation of free protoscolexes in hydatid fluid. They consist of a proligeral membrane and a cuticular layer, and bud off to form numerous protoscolexes.
- Exogenous daughter vesicles: these originate from proligeric membrane fragments embedded in the cuticle, which vesiculate, surround themselves with a cuticle, and form proto-scolexes.

- Hydatid fluid: this is a clear liquid, typically "rock water", in which the daughter vesicles are bathed. It is salty and hypertensive. It keeps the cyst under tension.

- The increase in fluid volume leads to an increase in cyst volume.

- Hydatid sand: this forms the sediment in the sloping part of the cyst. It is composed of proto-scolexes detached from the proligeral membrane or released from the vesicles, dehiscent capsules, daughter vesicles and hooks from degenerated and destroyed scolexes.

X- Natural history and complications :

Hydatid cysts develop very slowly, over several years. The myocardium is inelastic and resists cyst expansion, which explains why cardiac cysts grow more slowly than pulmonary cysts.

As a result, they may remain clinically inapparent for a long time, or be discovered by chance during a complication.

These complications may be due to compression of the coronary arteries, conduction pathways or valves.

Rupture, anaphylactic shock, embolization and superinfection are also possible complications. They can be life-threatening.

1. Fracture and cracking (80):

The rupture may involve the endo-cyst alone, or the endo-cyst and pericyst. Two types of rupture can be distinguished:

- **Rupture of the endocyst or fissuring:** This only involves the endocyst, while the pericyst remains intact.

These are fissures that allow fluid to pass into a virtual space between the pericyst and the endocyst. The latter collapses, but the cyst retains its size and appears macroscopically normal. It may progress to rupture.

It is favored by external stresses that weaken the cyst, notably the resistance of myocardial tissue to cyst expansion and the trauma generated by cardiac movements (62).

- **Complete rupture:** Rupture is a fatal medical-surgical emergency (81). The solution of continuity involves both the endocyst and the pericyst. It can occur as a result of direct or indirect trauma, after physical exertion, or spontaneously without any triggering factor.

What's more, as the cyst increases in size, intra-cystic pressure rises and the cyst will be under tension and may rupture at the slightest trigger (80).

- **Intracavitary rupture:** given the low-pressure regime prevailing in the right cavities, hydatid cyst development is usually subendocardial in right heart locations, which explains the possibility of intracavitary rupture (45). This rupture may be immediately fatal due to anaphylactic shock, or obstruction of a valvular orifice (82) (81).

In the right heart, it can also lead to hydatid pulmonary embolism. In the left heart, it can lead to systemic hydatid embolism.

Intracavitary rupture can also lead to hydatid metastases: hydatid material can disseminate through the small or large circulation, depending on the location of the cardiac hydatid cyst, resulting either in pulmonary seeding, or secondary localizations that can affect all organs (28).

The most frequent metastases are to the brain, and can result in intracranial hypertension, seizures and neurological deficits (48).

Di Bello et al (83) reported 104 cases of cysts complicated by intracavitary rupture, 91 of which were located in the right ventricle.

- **Intra-pericardial rupture:** this is the most frequent complication of left ventricular cysts, due to the frequency of sub-epicardial localization (45).

It can lead to acute pericarditis, with chest pain, dyspnea, palpitations and pericardial friction (29). The major risk is the occurrence of tamponade or constriction secondary to chronic pericardial effusion (82).

There are several types of pericarditis with effusion (84):

- Hydatido-pericardium: except in the case of compressive phenomena, this effusion may have no clinical significance. It results from the evolution of daughter vesicles in the pericardium after rupture of the subepicardial cyst into the pericardial cavity.

- Cardio-pericardial polycystic disease: primary grafting of one or more cysts onto the pericardium without associated cardiac involvement (4).

- **Intra-myocardial rupture:** this is responsible for local echinococcosis with a characteristic clustered appearance. (85).

2. Anaphylactic shock (86):

This is the most dreaded complication, as it is relatively frequent after cyst rupture, unpredictable and rapidly fatal.

Clinical signs may be sudden or progressive in onset. They are dominated by mucocutaneous signs (pruritus, urticaria, edema, etc.), respiratory signs (dyspnea, cough, bronchospasm, respiratory arrest, etc.), cardiovascular signs (tachycardia, hypotension, etc.) and digestive signs (nausea, vomiting, abdominal pain, etc.).

Anaphylactic reactions can take on many forms, ranging in severity from simple urticaria or isolated erythema to cardio-respiratory arrest.

During surgical treatment of cysts, the diagnosis of anaphylactic shock must be strongly suspected in the event of circulatory failure or collapse not explained by intraoperative bleeding, especially when associated with other clinical signs suggestive of an allergic mechanism, such as bronchospasm or cutaneous signs.

3. Embolisms:

The cardiac hydatid cyst grows over time and may present as a peripheral, cerebral or pulmonary embolization.

- Hydatid pulmonary embolism (87) Hydatid pulmonary embolism is caused by the seeding of daughter vesicles into the pulmonary circulation. Its starting point is usually a hydatid cyst of the right heart, particularly the right ventricle (42) (87) (41) (50).

Parasitic emboli can obstruct arterial vessels, leading to the development of pulmonary hypertension (88). They may give rise to secondary hydatid lesions responsible for destruction of the pulmonary parenchyma (89). These phenomena will later lead to chronic respiratory failure and chronic pulmonary heart disease.

The clinical signs of hydatid pulmonary embolism are polymorphous. The initial phase concomitant with cyst rupture is sometimes accompanied by anaphylactic shock or acute pulmonary heart disease, leading to sudden death. (42).

More often than not, this phase takes the form of febrile pneumonitis, or goes completely unnoticed. After a latency period of variable duration, hemoptysis, febrile pneumonitis and exertional dyspnea appear. (28) (50) (42).

The diagnosis of pulmonary embolism has benefited from the contribution of imaging.

Trans-thoracic echocardiography confirms the presence of a cyst in the right heart chambers.

Helical CT and MRI confirm the diagnosis of pulmonary embolism, provide additional information on the location and morphology of the cyst, and verify the existence of any other extra-thoracic localizations (87) (39).

The prognosis for hydatid pulmonary embolism remains poor. It is often discovered at autopsy.

Embolism is due to purely mechanical obstruction of the pulmonary artery by cysts and daughter vesicles. (49).

- **Systemic embolisms:** They can be :

- Cerebral embolisms causing ischemic stroke with neurological deficit.

Byard and Bourne (13) reported the case of a 12-year-old boy who died following rupture of a left ventricular hydatid cyst complicated by cerebral arterial embolism.

- Arterial embolisms of the lower limbs with acute ischemia and gangrene.

- Renal, splenic, coronary or other embolisms...

4. Mechanical complications :

They occur when the cyst reaches a certain volume and comes into contact with neighbouring structures.

Whatever the mechanism of mechanical complications, whether related to compression or obstruction, the cyst may be responsible for right or left congestive heart failure, or congestive heart failure overall.

- **Valvular obstruction:** This is the result of two different mechanisms linked to the compression or obstruction exerted by the cyst:

- Obstruction: narrowing of the valve orifice by a large cyst protruding into one of the heart chambers (figure 12) (90).

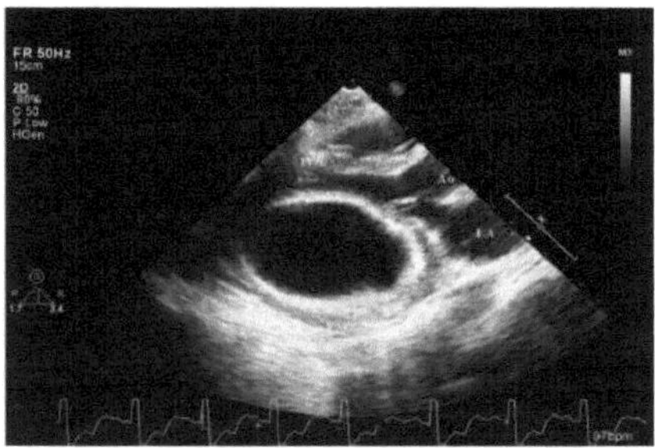

Figure 12: Very large left ventricular cyst causing mitral and aortic valve obstruction (90).

- Compression: leading to valvular insufficiency through adhesion or retraction of the leaflets to the adjacent wall of a cyst.

The symptomatology secondary to these dysfunctions is highly polymorphic, and depends on which valve is affected.

- **Coronary artery compression:** extrinsic compression of coronary arteries by cysts can disrupt myocardial perfusion, manifesting as angina-like chest pain and electrical signs typical of myocardial ischemia (81) (44).

5. Rhythm and conduction disorders :

These disorders result from compression of the surrounding conduction tissue and myocardium by the cyst (91).

- **Conductive disorders:** These disorders may be complete atrioventricular block, bundle-branch block, or atrial fibrillation. (92).

These disorders may be reversible after surgical or medical treatment. Interventricular septal cysts can frequently disrupt conduction pathways and lead to conductive disorders (92). Thus, lipothymic or syncopal malaise may be the mode of revelation of an interventricular septal cyst (48).

- **Rhythm disorders:** supraventricular or ventricular rhythm disorders may complicate cysts of the interventricular septum or free wall of the heart (56). A case of apical hydatid cyst complicated by ventricular tachycardia in a young 24-year-old patient was described by a Tunisian team in 2014 (93). A transition to sustained ventricular tachycardia can be fatal, with a risk of sudden death.

6. Infection :

Infection of the cystic contents may remain latent, manifesting itself as a slight rise in temperature, or it may manifest itself as systemic manifestations, such as fever with chills, altered general condition, hyperleukocytosis... The risk of progression to septicemia or even septic shock is significant. (6) (61).

7. Sudden death:

Sudden death due to cardiac hydatid cysts is a rare entity with little documentation in the literature. It may be the inaugural complication (45). In most cases, it is preceded by prodromal clinical signs that are variable and non-specific: abdominal pain, chest pain, dyspnea...

The leading causes of sudden death from hydatid cysts are anaphylactic shock, followed by valve obstruction, infection and hydatid pulmonary embolism.

8. Involution:

In 12% of cases, spontaneous evolution may lead to healing with involution of the cyst. Its contents become thickened, often leading to the formation of calcifications (55).

Calcifications of the cyst are important to note, as they are pathognomonic of cardiac hydatidosis (55).

XI- Differential diagnosis :

1. Cardiac tumors (94) :

Echocardiography offers excellent sensitivity for the diagnosis of hydatid cysts. However, some cysts have a solid appearance on echocardiography, posing the problem of differential diagnosis with primary or secondary tumors of the heart.

This aspect is explained by degenerative or infectious phenomena (61).

2. Infective endocarditis :

Unlike hydatid cysts, vegetations affect valve structures, and can lead to mutilation. They often occur on valves that are already diseased. Endocarditis lesions are also characterized by their mobility.

Walpot et al (95) reported the case of a patient with endocarditis affecting the mitral valve in the form of hyperechoic vegetation surrounded by anechoic fluid simulating a hydatid cyst (figure 13).

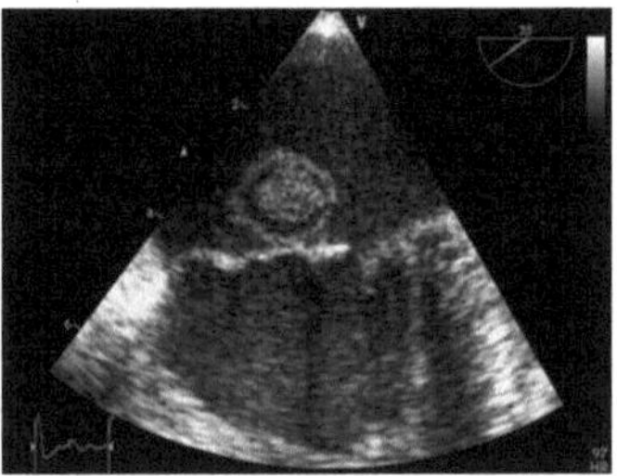

Figure 13: Sonographic appearance of mitral valve vegetation (95).

3. Thrombus :

Thrombus is a differential diagnosis with hydatid cyst when it develops at the expense of a cardiac cavity.

The common complication is the possibility of peripheral embolism.

Thrombi often develop in the setting of severe heart failure. Treatment is heparin therapy, followed by anti-vitamin K drugs.

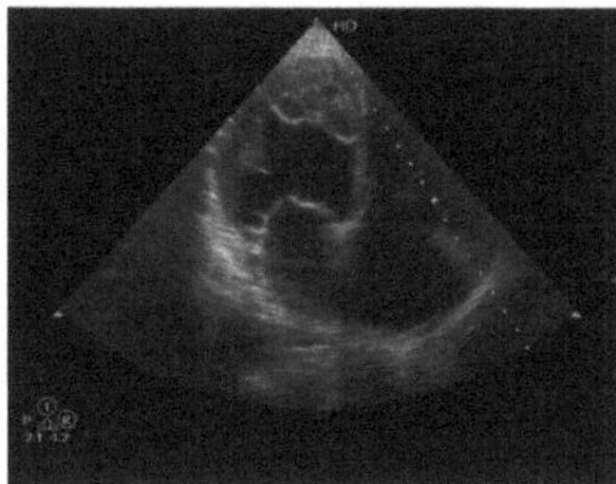

Figure 14: Image of left apical thrombus (96).

4. Ventricular aneurysm :

Hydatid cysts can mimic left ventricular aneurysms, especially in the calcification stage.

The existence of other cystic localizations, whether or not associated with positive serology, helps to guide the diagnosis, which can sometimes be ambiguous.

It is easily diagnosed by angiography (97).

XII- Treatment :

Once the diagnosis has been confirmed, the severity of possible complications calls for rapid therapeutic management.

Radical treatment is surgical excision, as cardiac hydatidosis is fatal sooner or later.

The information provided by imaging is a great help in the surgical approach.

1. Medical treatment :

Medical treatment is a complementary and adjuvant therapy to surgery for the eradication of cardiac hydatidosis.

Drugs belonging to the benzimidazole class appear to be the most effective in the medical treatment of hydatid disease.

Among benzimidazoles, albendazole is the most effective. It reduces cyst size, parasite viability and the frequency of post-operative recurrence (41) (98).

It is used at a dose of 10 to 15 mg/kg per day in courses spaced 15 days apart for six months (92) (65).

Biological monitoring is essential throughout treatment with albendazole (99) . It includes :

- Transaminase levels should be measured before starting treatment, every two weeks for the first month, then once a month for the following two months, and quarterly after the third month of treatment.

- Blood count at the same rate.

- There are no specific contraindications to prescribing albendazole.

Isolated medical treatment is indicated for patients who cannot undergo surgery because of the presence of too many hydatid cysts affecting several organs, or because of a debilitated patient. (65) (100).

2. Surgical treatment :

2. 1 General :

The intervention must enable :

- Perform a complete cyst resection.

- Good parietal repair.

- Perform a thorough exploration of the heart in search of another location.

- Minimize the risk of intra-operative parasite dissemination, which is always possible during surgery, and which can lead to the development of secondary metastatic echinococcosis.

2. 2. Approach :

- **Sternotomy:** The classic approach currently used by most surgeons is the median sternotomy. It enables rapid and easy installation of the CEC, and tumour removal under optimum conditions, by allowing access to all four cavities (figure 15).

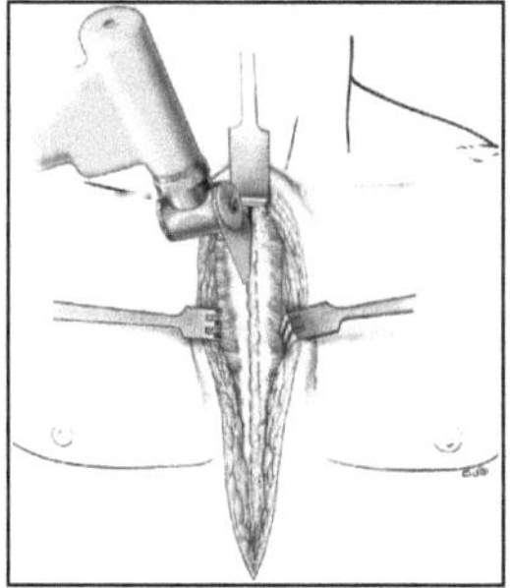

Figure 15: Vertical median sternotomy (101).

- **Mini-sternotomy:** This technique offers a more aesthetic scar, rapid mobilization and a shorter hospital stay. It also reduces the risk of surgical wound infection (Fig. 16).

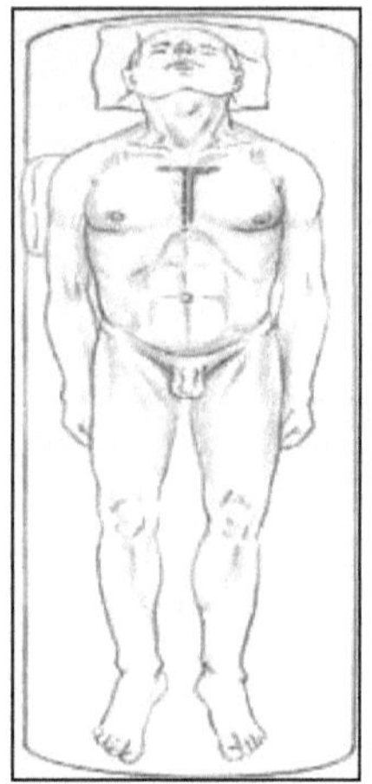

Figure 16: Inverted L- or T-shaped mini-sternotomy (102).

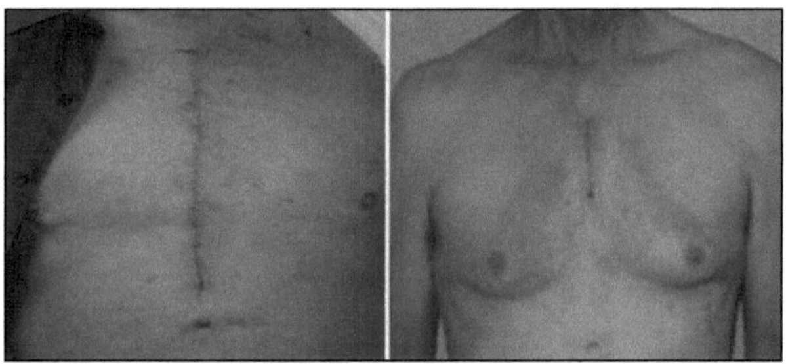

Figure 17: Cutaneous scar from median sternotomy (left) and mini-sternotomy (right).

- **Posterolateral thoracotomy:** Can be used for pericardial hydatid cysts. It is particularly useful for the simultaneous treatment of pulmonary hydatid cysts.

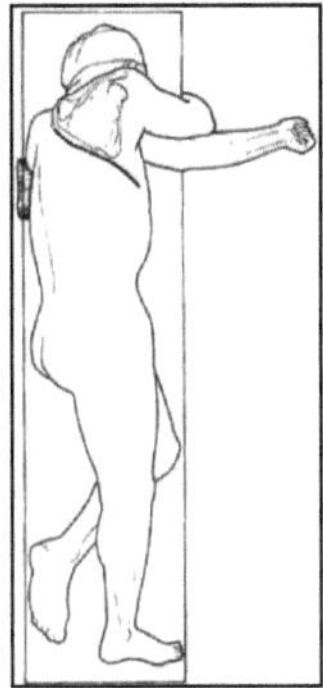

Figure 18: Posterolateral thoracotomy (103).

- **Right anterolateral thoracotomy:** This approach can be used for surgery on a hydatid cyst in the right or left atrium. It has an aesthetic advantage, especially for women.

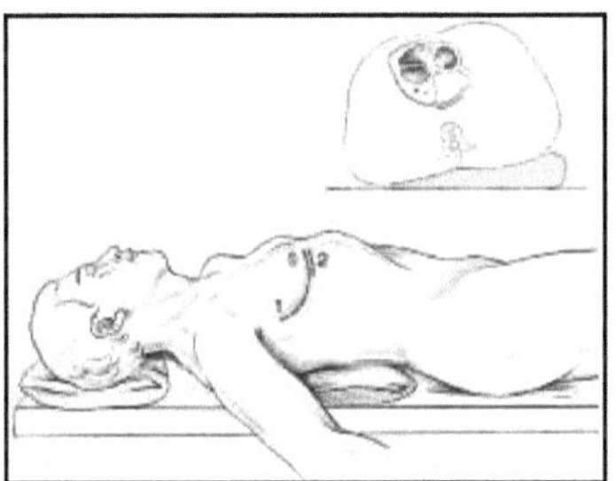

Figure 19: Right anterolateral thoracotomy (102).

2. 3 Video surgery :

Intra-thoracic endoscopic techniques have been practiced for a long time, but cardiac endoscopic surgery began in the 90s and was initially dedicated to valvular and then coronary surgery (104).

Cardiac surgery is moving towards a totally endoscopic approach, in order to reduce scar size, healing time and hospitalization.

In this case, instruments are introduced via trocars with a diameter of around 10 mm. It may or may not be combined with an anterolateral thoracotomy.

This technique is very difficult because the surgeon no longer has a direct view of the surgical site, and requires a slower learning curve.
It is not well suited to the surgical treatment of cardiac hydatid cysts, due to the greater risk of dissemination.

2.4 Extracorporeal circulation :

Surgical treatment of intracardiac cysts is generally performed under bypass grafting, to obtain a bloodless surgical field and an immobile heart, for radical surgical treatment while avoiding contamination by cyst contents.

- **Principle:** CEC provides temporary circulatory and respiratory support during surgery:

- Circulatory function: via a pump ensuring perfusion flow and pressure.

- Respiratory function: via an oxygenator providing oxygen and extracting carbon monoxide.
Under certain flow (2.4 to 2.6l/min/m2 body surface area at 37°) and pressure (above 60 mm Hg) conditions, venous blood is diverted from the right heart inlet (right atrium or both vena cava) and reinjected with oxygen at the left heart outlet (ascending aorta), to ensure satisfactory tissue oxygenation (figures 20 and 21).

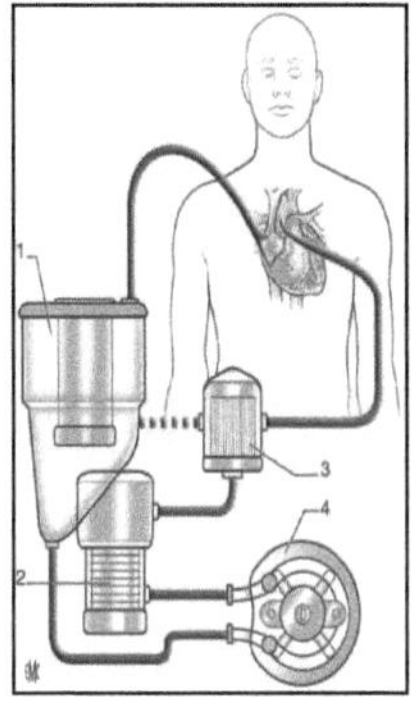

1. Cardiotomy reservoir; 2. Oxygenator; 3. Arterial filter;

4. Roller pump (105).

Figure 20: Classic extracorporeal circulation circuit.

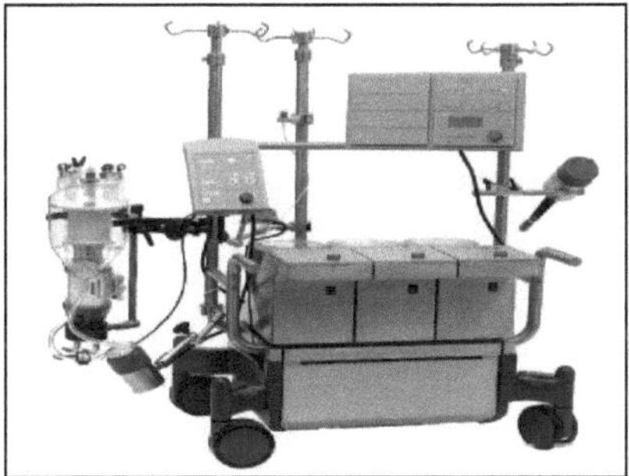

Figure 21: Extracorporeal circulation equipment (105).

Aspiration of blood from the surgical field during cyst resection and reinjection into the pump is controversial, given the risk of intraoperative dissemination of daughter vesicles.

Some authors recommend clamping the pulmonary artery during bypass surgery to avoid pulmonary hydatid embolization in cases of right-heart cysts. (1) (12).

2.5 Myocardial protection :

To achieve an immobile, bloodless heart, coronary circulation must be interrupted, and myocardial protection must be ensured, essentially by injecting cardioplegic fluid into the coronary network.

The heart can be stopped in normothermia by injecting a warm cardioplegia solution into the aortic root at the moment of aortic clamping, followed by repeated doses every 15 minutes.

It can also be performed in moderate hypothermia by injecting a cold cardioplegia solution at the root of the aorta at the moment of aortic clamping, followed by repeated doses every 15 minutes.

2.6 Beating heart surgery :

Beating heart surgery involves operating on a heart that continues to beat, thus avoiding the need for bypass surgery. It offers a lower risk of post-operative atrial fibrillation, fewer blood transfusions, and a lower risk of post-CEC cognitive impairment, with a shorter hospital stay (106) (107).

It is indicated in cases of hydatid cysts developed on the sub-epicardial side and without communication with the cardiac cavities. (108).

2.7 Cyst exposure routes :

The choice of approach must take into account the size, location and number of cysts. The best approach should :

- Allow minimal manipulation of the cyst.

- Provide adequate exposure to ensure complete cystic resection.

- Allowing inspection of all four heart chambers.

- This minimizes the risk of recurrence.

Several routes have been proposed for approaching and extracting the cyst:

- **Right auriculotomy:** This approach is used for cysts developed in the right atrium, inter-atrial septum or even right ventricular cysts (figure 22).

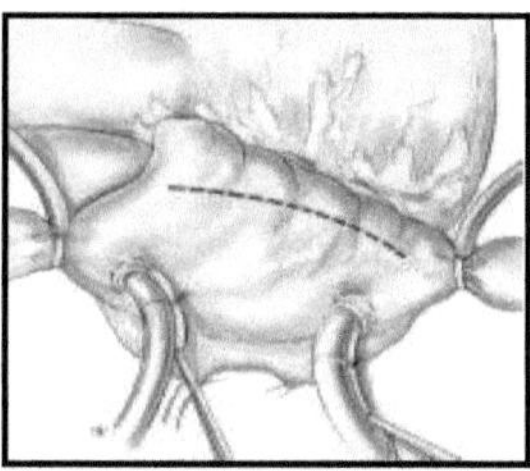

Figure 22: Right auriculotomy (109).

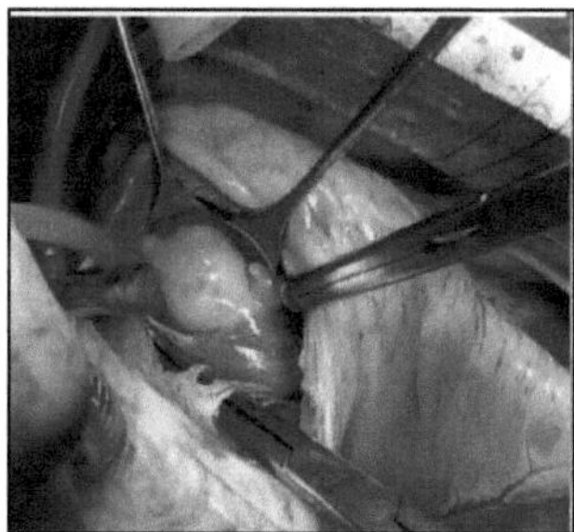

Figure 23: Resection of a cyst through a right auriculotomy (110).

- **Left auriculotomy: used for** surgery on hydatid cysts developing within the left auricle.

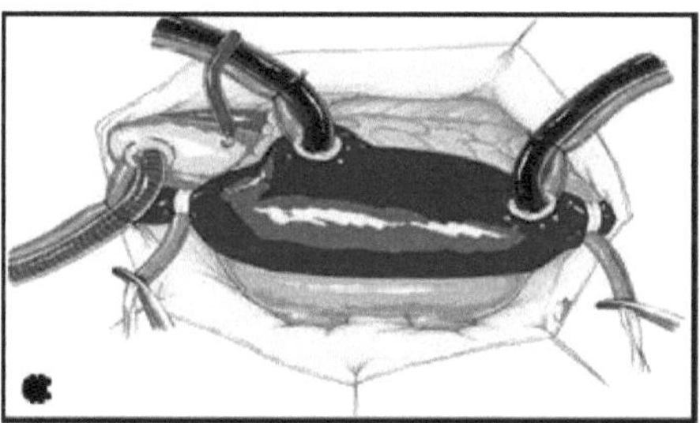

Figure 24: Left auriculotomy in Sondergaardt sulcus (111).

- **Right ventriculotomy:** The ventricular incision is used in cases of cystic localization in the free wall of the right ventricle. The location of the ventriculotomy depends on the location of the cyst (Fig. 25).

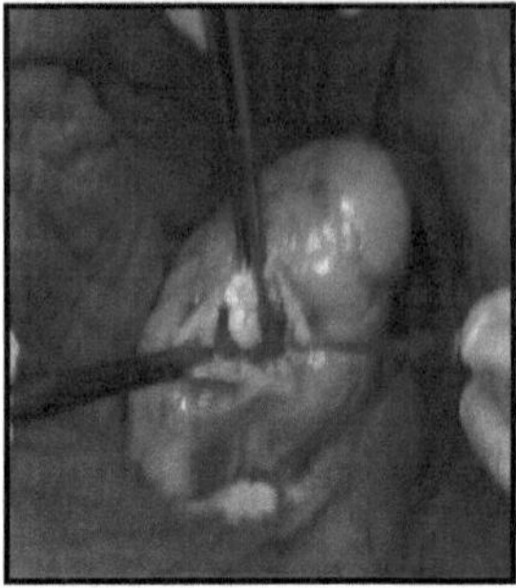

Figure 25: Intraoperative view showing excision of a cyst from the wall of the ventricle doit (112).

- **Left ventriculotomy:**

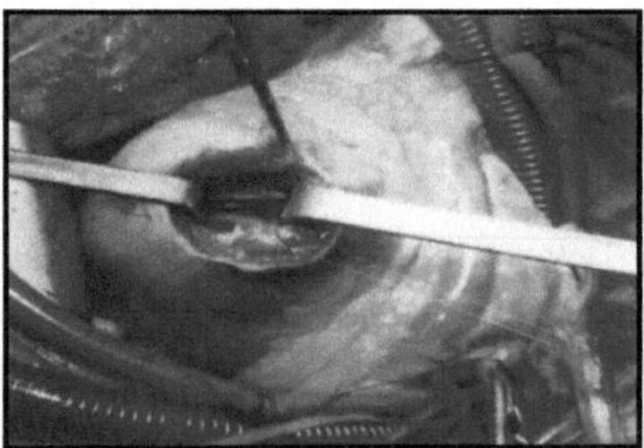

Figure 26: Intraoperative view after resection of a ventricular wall cyst through a left ventriculotomy (12).

2. 8. cyst resection: cysto-peri-cystectomy :

It is the best surgical procedure when feasible.

Before resecting the cyst, macroscopic exploration of the pericardium and heart walls is necessary.

A cyst with parietal development is a smooth, whitish formation protruding into the corresponding wall (figure no. 27).

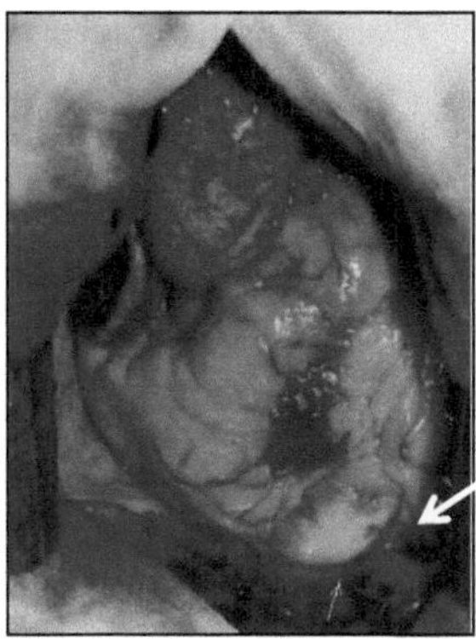

Figure 27: Intraoperative view showing the macroscopic appearance of a hydatid cyst in the wall of the left ventricle (arrow). (31).

The first step is rigorous protection of the surrounding tissue with hypertonic saline compresses around the cyst to protect the ventricles. (113).

In order to sterilize the parasite prior to extraction, and to avoid any intraoperative secondary dissemination, the hydatid fluid is punctured in the middle of the cyst using a trocar, and hypertonic serum is injected. When the cyst is unilocular, it collapses immediately (33).

Pericystectomy involves resection of the fibrous scar tissue, with varying degrees of sclerosis. It should be as economical as possible (figure 28).

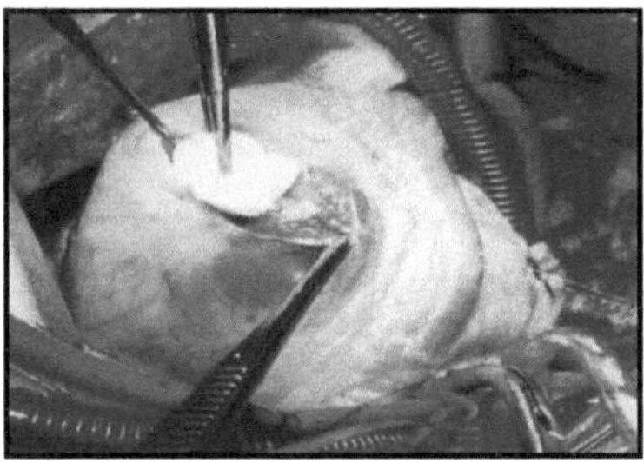

Figure 28: Intraoperative view showing resection of cystic material through the ventriculotomy (11).

When total pericystectomy is not feasible, a partial pericystectomy may be performed to preserve proper function of the cavity concerned (114).

The entire hydatid membrane is removed (figure 29).

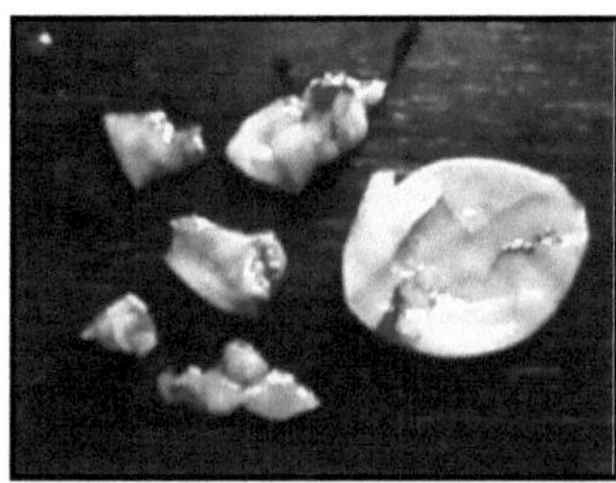

Figure 29: Macroscopic appearance of removed hydatid membranes (4).

2. 9. repair of the defect resulting from resection (1) (12) (31) :

After resection of ventricular wall cysts, loss of substance may be significant and may require patch plasty (figure 30).

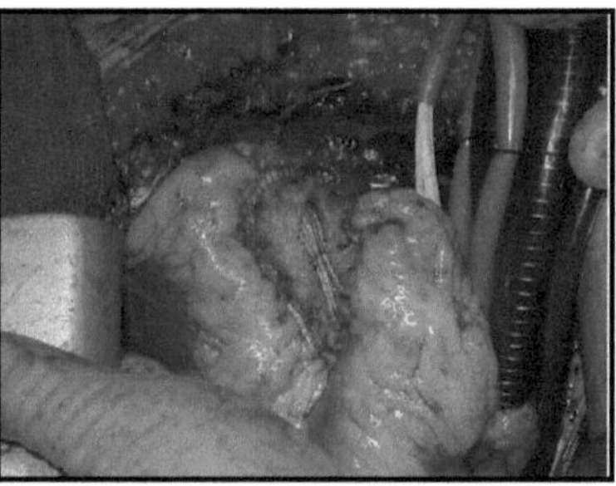

Figure 30: Intraoperative view showing ventriculotomy closure with a prosthetic patch (31).

In the case of SIV cysts, septal dysfunction may sometimes require plasty and reinforcement with Teflon splints. The integrity of the septum must always be checked after cyst resection.

2. 10. Related gestures :

- **Associated valve surgery:** The cyst has been described to adhere to valve tissue. After cystectomy, this may necessitate valve plasty or, exceptionally, valve replacement. (115).

Apaydin et al (116) described the case of a patient with a cyst on a mitral valve pillar responsible for severe mitral insufficiency treated by resection of the cyst with mitral plasty.

A hydatid localization in the right ventricle with invasion of the posterior pillar of the tricuspid valve was described by Sensoz Y et al. (31) (117). It required resection of the cyst carrying the tricuspid valve through a right ventriculotomy, and replacement of the valve by bioprosthesis.

- **Associated coronary bypass:** Large cysts and numerous cysts, by affecting a large part of the myocardium, are likely to have a significant functional impact (118). Their surgical resection will therefore remove a large part of the myocardium.

Tencer et al (23) in their series of 13 patients operated on for intra-cardiac hydatid cysts, reported the case of a patient operated on for a left atrial cyst by left atrial bypass associated with aorto-coronary bypass and myocardial bridge resection.

Sirlak M et al (118) reported the case of a patient with two cysts in the apical wall of the left ventricle. During resection of the cysts, one marginal was sacrificed necessitating bypass surgery via the left internal mammary artery on the marginal (figure no. 31).

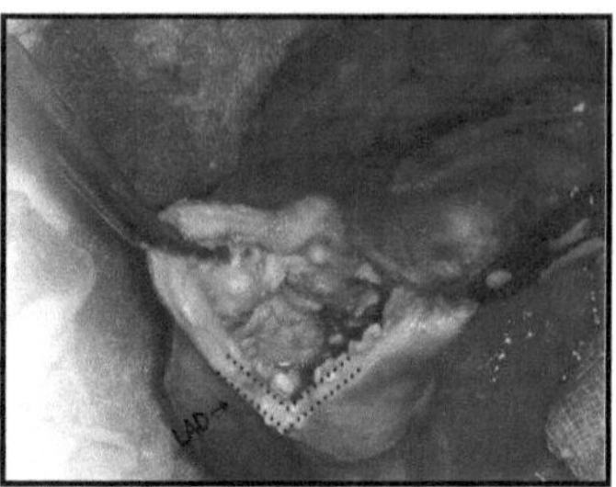

Figure 31: Intraoperative photograph showing sectioning of the margin during opening of the hydatid cyst (118).

2. 11. In case of multiple cardiac hydatidosis :

Cases of multiple intracardiac hydatid cysts have been described in the literature. The discovery may be made preoperatively by imaging techniques or by intraoperative macroscopic exploration.

Surgical resection of all lesions leads to a more prolonged procedure, with a higher complication rate.

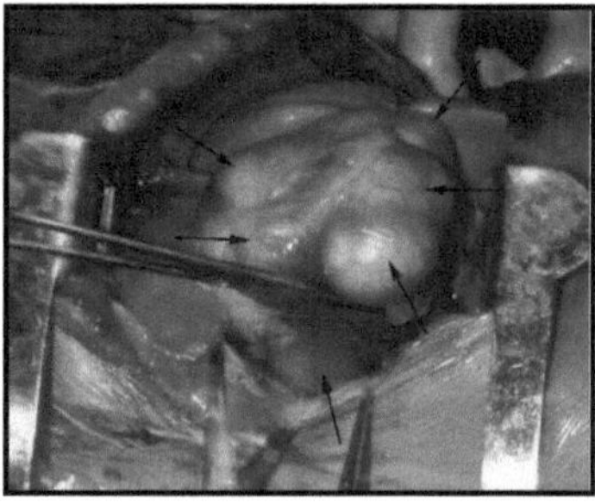

Figure 32: Intraoperative image of multiple hydatid cysts (119).

2. 12. The end of the intervention :

This is the stage that involves checking the integrity of the heart's cavities. Careful washing of the cavities is essential.

After suturing the access ports, purging the left cavities, declamping, warming up, and after the heart's rhythm has returned (spontaneously or by defibrillation), bypass surgery is gradually stopped if the heart's hemodynamic state allows.

Finally, the surgeon closes the thorax, after pericardial and mediastinal drainage.

2. 13. In case of associated pulmonary hydatidosis :

Unilateral or bilateral pulmonary hydatidosis is rare. It justifies resection at the same time as heart cyst surgery. (112). Sternotomy offers good exposure of the heart and both lungs, and is less likely to cause post-operative pain than two-stage surgery with sternotomy and thoracotomy.

What's more, combined surgery means shorter hospital stays and lower treatment costs.

XIII- Therapeutic results :

1. Early postoperative results:

- **Operative mortality:** Hydatid cyst surgery is a low-risk operation.

Mortality ranges from 0.1 to 0.25% according to the literature (8). Mortality is related to complications of the surgical procedure, such as ventricular rupture, ventricular arrhythmias, peripheral embolism, or cyst rupture leading to anaphylactic shock (120).

- **Early post-operative complications:** Conduction pathway damage during septal cyst resection is common. The result is post-operative atrioventricular block, which may require permanent electro-systolic pacing with a pacemaker (121).

Early deaths have been reported in the literature following mechanical complications such as rupture of the interventricular septum after resection of a hydatid cyst at this level (122).

2. Late postoperative results:

After the operation, clinical, biological, radiological and ultrasound monitoring is essential to detect any recurrence (58).

Late mortality after surgical treatment is 4.8% (123). Mortality may occur as a result of abnormal cardiac structures or ventricular rhythm disturbances on surgical scars.

Cases of recurrence of cardiac hydatid cysts have been reported in the literature (Table III) (124).

Table III: Cases of cardiac hydatid recurrence reported in the literature.

Study duration/country	Number of patients	Average age (years)	Heart disease	Extra-cardiac	Treatment and progress

52

			Gender (% women)		damage (%)	
Dali 2000 (64)	1988/1998 Tunisia	17	33/47 %	Myocardium Pericardium	70.5	17 operated 3 deaths
Thameur 2000 (33)	1970/1997 Tunisia	45	-	-	33.3	45 operated 2 deaths 2 recurrences
Khaldoun 2003 (47)	1983/2001 Tunisia	14	27.7	Myocardium Pericardium	57.1	-
Akar 2003 (120)	1984/2001 Turkey	12	31 33.33%	Myocardium		12 operated 3 deaths
Jerbi 2004 (125)	1991/2003 Tunisia	19	30 52.6%	-	-	19 operated 1 death
Bouraoui 2005 (126)	1985/2001 Tunisia	12	40 83.3%	Myocardium Pericardium	-	-
Elhattaoui 2006 (25)	1999/2005 Morocco	10	24.7 40%	Myocardium Pericardium	70	7 operated 2 albendazole 2 deaths
Orhan 2007 (1)	1967/2006 Turkey	25	31 68%	Myocardium Pericardium Multiple	28	25 operated 1 death 1 repeat offence
Murat 2007 (124)	1978/2002 China	15	23 40 %	Myocardium Pericardium	0	15 operated 1 death 4 recurrences
Kabbani 2007 (127)	1989-2005 Syria	19	25.6 57.9%	Myocardium Pericardium	63.2	19 operated
Tasdemir 2009 (128)	1982/2007 Turkey	10	39 20 %	Myocardium Pericardium	10	10 operated 2 recurrences
Molavipour 2010 (129)	1992/2004 Iran	11	25.6 57.9%	Myocardium Multiple		11 operated 1 death
Tuncer 2010 (23)	1991/2009 Turkey	13	36 46.2 %	Myocardium	61.5	13 operated 1 recurrence

XIV- Conclusion :

Human hydatidosis is a cosmopolitan disease caused by the development in humans of the larval form of the taenia Echinococcus granulosus. It remains a public health problem in Tunisia, as well as in many other parts of the world.

Hydatid localization in the heart is rare. It is characterized by its long clinical latency and unpredictable course, which can be marked by a number of complications, the most serious of which is sudden death.

Clinical signs may include atypical precordialgia, typical anginal pain, rhythm disturbances such as extrasystoles or ventricular tachycardia, lipothymia secondary to third-degree atrioventricular block in cysts located at the interventricular septum, hemoptysis, cough in association with accompanying lung damage, epigastralgia, and altered general condition in association with advanced polyvisceral involvement.

Allergic manifestations can be the only clinical symptomatology, ranging from focal urticarial crises to full-blown anaphylactic shock, which can be fatal from the outset. They are a sign of severity, reflecting the phenomenon of cyst fissuring, with the release of hydatid fluid.

Echocardiography, computed tomography (CT) and magnetic resonance imaging (MRI) make a considerable contribution to positive diagnosis.

Similarly, immunological and pharmacological tests are important for diagnosis, particularly hydatid serology, which is essential both for diagnostic purposes and for post-treatment monitoring.

Treatment is surgical, as spontaneous evolution is fatal in the short or long term. Medical treatment is only conceivable as a complement.

Surgical treatment involves a precise open-chest lesion assessment, cystectomy or at least emptying of the cyst, which is sterilized by intra-cystic injection of a hypertonic parasiticide solution, while respecting the myocardium.

Mortality, which used to be high, has fallen with diagnostic advances in imaging and therapeutic advances in surgical techniques.

In most series, the average age of patients is between 30 and 40 years. In several publications, the frequency was higher for males.

The clinical presentation is polymorphous and unspecific. It varies according to the size of the cyst, its stage of development, its location in relation to the valve orifices and conduction tissue, and its location in the right or left heart.

They may manifest as dyspnea, chest pain, palpitations, syncope, general signs, allergic manifestations or embolic complications, or they may be asymptomatic and be discovered by chance.

Cysts developing in the left heart may be complicated by systemic embolism in the brain, aorta, kidneys, spleen, coronary arteries or arteries of the lower limbs, leading to ischemic accidents. Cysts developing in the right heart may be complicated by pulmonary embolism.

The main advantage of these polymorphous signs is that they prompt a request for a cardiac ultrasound scan, which will most often establish the diagnosis. Thus, TTE is most often used to establish a positive diagnosis, to specify the size and appearance of the cyst, and the hemodynamic repercussions, in order to guide the therapeutic approach. TEE can be used to visualize small cysts that cannot be seen on TTE, and to study the condition of the valves and the extent of valve leakage.

The main advantage of CT is that it can be used to assess extension to adjacent structures through thoracoabdominal acquisition, in search of multi-visceral localization.

MRI can also be used to assess mediastinal extension and look for other liver, spleen and kidney sites.

Hydatid serology is always essential for both diagnostic and post-therapeutic purposes, to assess the efficacy of treatment. ELISA and indirect immunofluorescence are the most sensitive tests. Immunoelectrophoresis is the most specific test.

Rupture, anaphylactic shock, valvular obstruction, coronary artery compression, embolization, rhythm and conduction disorders, and superinfection are possible complications during the natural course of cardiopericardial hydatidosis. They can be life-threatening.

Once the diagnosis has been confirmed, the severity of these complications calls for rapid therapeutic management, based essentially on surgical removal of the cyst. Medical treatment is an adjuvant to surgery.

The aim of surgery is to achieve complete resection of the cyst, good repair of the resulting parietal defect, and good exploration of the heart in search of another location, while minimizing the risk of parasite dissemination intraoperatively. The classic approach is the median sternotomy.

The short-term prognosis of these procedures is good, with a mortality rate of between 0.1 and 0.25 according to the literature. Long-term prognosis is dominated by the risk of hydatid recurrence. Regular ultrasound and serological monitoring is therefore essential.

Eradicating hydatid disease in endemic countries requires effective individual and collective prevention. Any prophylaxis program must aim to interrupt the natural biological cycle of *Echinococcus Granulosus, which* evolves in dogs and sheep, or at least to interrupt its access to humans.

Health education is one of the fundamental components of any action to combat hydatidosis. It involves informing the population at risk, particularly the rural population, about hydatid cysts, their severity and transmission cycle, and the preventive and control measures that individuals and families can take to avoid becoming infested.

On an individual level, general hygiene measures are an important part of prevention:

- Personal hygiene, especially hand hygiene before preparing and eating food, and thorough washing of fruits and vegetables.
- Careful washing of raw food that may have been contaminated by dog excrement.
- Avoid promiscuity between humans and dogs likely to be parasitized.

Bibliography :

1. Orhan G, Ozay B, Tartan Z, Kurc E, Ketenci B, Sargin M et al. *Cardiac hydatid cyst surgery: thirty-nine years of experience.* Annals of cardiology and angiology 2008: 57; 58-61.
2. Chaouachi B, Ben Salah S, Lakhoua R, Hammou A, Gharbi H.A, Saied H. *Hydatid cysts in children: diagnostic and therapeutic aspects: about 1195 cases .* Annales de pédiatrie 1989 : 36 ; 441-9.
3. Oudni Mrad M, Mrad S, Gorcii M, Mekki M, Belguith M, Harrabi I et al. *Childhood hydatid echinococcosis in Tunisia: Fertility and cyst localization.* Bull Soc Pathol Exot 2007: 100; 1: 10-13.
4. Elkarimia S, Ouldelgadiab N, Gacema H, Zouizrab Z, Boumzebrab D, Blelaabidiac B, Elhattaouia M. *Tamponnade revealing an intrapericardial hydatid cyst: a case report.* Annales de Cardiologie et d'Angéiologie 63 (2014) 267-270.
5. P, Aubry. *Hydatidosis-Echinococcosis-Hydatid cyst.* Tropical medicine 2003.
6. Sakhri J, Ben Ali A. *The hydatid cyst of the liver.* J Chir 2004 : 141 ; 381-9.
7. Brechignac X, Durieu I, Perinetti M, Geriniere C, Richalet D. *Hydatid cyst of the heart.* La presse médicale, avril, 1997, n°26, 663-665.
8. Pasaoglu I, Dogan R, Hazan E, Oram A, Bozer AY. *Right ventricular hydatid cyst causing recurrent pulmonary emboli.* Eur J Cardiothorac Surg. 1992;6:161-163.
9. Amrani M, Zouaidia F, Belabbas MA. *Hydatidosis: about some unusual localizations.* Médecine Tropicale 2000, 60, 271-273.
10. Tellez G, Nojek C, Juffe A, Rufilanchas J, O'Connor F, Figuera D. *Cardiac echinococcosis: report of 3 cases and review of the literature.* Ann Thorac Surg 1976; 21: 425-30.
11. Artucio H, Reglia JL, Di Bello R, et al. *Hydatid cyst of the interventricular septum of the heart ruptured into the right ventricle: first case in the world literature diagnosed and successfully operated upon with open heart surgery.* J Thorac Cardiovasc S.
12. Mehmet Kaplan, Murat Demirtas, Serdar Cimen, and Azmi Ozler. *Cardiac hydatid cysts with intracavitary expansion.* Ann Thorac Surg 2001; 71: 1587-90.
13. Byard R.W, Bourne A.J. *Cardiac echinococcosis with fatal intracerebral embolism.* Arch Dis Child 1991: 66; 155-6.
14. Budke C, Deplazes P, Torgerson P.R. *Global socioeconomic impact of cystic echinococcosis.* Emerg Infect Dis 2006: 12; 296-303.

15. Athanassiadi K, Kalavrouziotis G, Loutsidis A, Bellenis I, Exarchos N. *Surgical treatment of echinococcosis by a transthoracic approach: a review of 85 cases.* European journal of cardio-thoracic surgery 1998: 14; 134-40.

16. Lagardère B, Chevallier B, Cheriet R. *Hydatid cyst of the child.* EMC éditions techniques, Pédiatrie 1995: 4; 350- B-10.

17. P, Aubry. *Hydatidosis or hydatid cyst: News 2009.* **Médecine** tropicale 2009.

18. M.K, Chahed. *Surgical incidence of hydatid cyst in Tunisia: Results of the 221-2005 survey and evolutionary trend between 1977-200.* Archives de l'institut Pasteur de Tunis 2010.

19. Kosecik M, Karaoglanoglu M, Yamak B. *Pericardial hydatid cyst presenting with cardiac tamponade.* Can J Cardiol 2006: 22; 145-7.

20. Yaliniz H, Tokcan A, Salih OK, Ulus T. *Surgical treatment of cardiac hydatid disease: a report of 7 cases.* Tex Heart Inst J 2006; 33: 333-9.

21. Minetto E, Prinotti C, Purini T. *Sudden death due to primary echinococcosis of the interatrial septum. Clinical and medico-legal interest.* Minerva Medicolegale 1964; 84: 189-94.

22. Cevirme D, Yerebalkan C, Bayrakatar S, Sunar H. *Cardiac hydatid cyst of the interatrial septum.* . Wien Med Wochenschr 2009; 159: 17-8.

23. Tuncer E, Tas SG, Mataraci I et al. *Surgical treatment of cardiac hydatid disease in 13 patients.* . Tex Heart Inst J 2010; 37: 189-93.

24. Nazim Kankilic; Mehmet Salih Aydin, Tansel Günendi, Mustafa Göz. Unusual Hydatid Cysts: Cardiac and Pelvic-Ilio-femoral Hydatid Cyst Case Reports and Literature Review. Braz J Cardiovasc Surg 2020;35(4):565-72.

25. Elhattaoui M, Charei N, Bennis A, Tahiri A, Chraibi N. *Hydatid cyst of the heart, about 10 cases.* Archive des maladies du cœur, 2006, n°99, 19-25.

26. Tetik O, Yetkin U, Yazıcı M, Tulukoglu E, Gurbuz A. *A case with giant hydatid cyst localized in right ventricle wall.* Turkish J Thorac Cardiovasc Surg. 2004; 12: 265-267.

27. Yuksel Besir, Arif Gucu, Suleyman Surer, Orhan Rodoplu, Mehmet Melek, Omer Tetik. *Giant cardiac hydatid cyst in the interventricular septum protruding to right ventricular epicardium.* Indian heart journal 6 5 (2 0 1 3) 8 1-8 3.

28. Jerbi S, Romdhani N, Tarmiz A, Kortas C, Mlika S, Khelil N et al. *Emboligenic hydatid cyst of the right heart.* Ann Cardiol Angéiol 2008: 57; 62-5.

29. Chellaoui M, Bouhouch R, Akjouj M, Chat L, Alami D. *Pericardial hydatidosis: about 3 observations.* Journal de Radiologie, 2003, 84, 329-331.

30. **Sabah I, Yacin F, Okay T.** *Rupture of presumed hydatid cyst of the interventricular septum diagnosed by transoesophageal echocardiography.* Heart, 1998, n°79, 420-421.

31. **Sensoz Y, Ozkokelib M, Atesa M, Akcara M.** *Right ventricle hydatid cyst requiring tricuspid valve excision.* International Journal of Cardiology 101 (2005) 339- 341.

32. **Aksakal E, Degirmenci H, Bakirci E M.** *A case of mitral valve involvement by hydatid cyst disease.* International Journal of Cardiology 140, Supplement 1 (2010) S1-S93.

33. **Thameur H, Abdelmoula S, Chenik S.** *Cardio pericardial hydatid cysts.* World Journal Surgery, 2001, 25, 58-67.

34. **Grozavu C, Ilias M, Pantile D.** *Multivisceral echinococcosis: concept, diagnosis, management.* Chirurgia (Bucur) 2014; 109 (6): 758-68.

35. **Yunfei Ling, Yongjuan Qian, Wei Meng, Ke Lin.** *Unusual cause of chest pain in a 13 year-old young child: Left ventricular hydatid cyst.* International Journal of Cardiology 174 (2014) 99-100.

36. **El** Boussaadani B, Regragui H, Bouhdadi H, Wazaren H, Ajhoun I, Laaroussi M, Cherti M. Primary cardiac hydatid cyst presenting with massive pericardial effusion: a case report. Egypt Heart J. 2020; 72(1): 51.

37. **Bouzidi A, Chehab F.** *Surgical treatment of bilio-cystic fistulas of hydatid origin: A propos de 83 cases.* J Chir 1997: 134; 114-8.

38. **Yilmaz N, Kizilca O, Demircan T, Karadas U, Kir M, Metin K, Ugurlu B, Unal N.** *Pulmonary Embolism due to Ruptured Giant Right Atrial Cyst Hydatid in a Child. .* The American Journal of Cardiology March 2014 13-16.

39. **Oliver J.M, Sotillo J.F, Dominquez F.J, Lopez De Sa E, Calvo L, Salvador A et al.** *Two-dimensional echocardiographic features of echinococcosis of the heart and great blood vessels. Clinical and surgical implications.* Circulation 1988: 78; 327-37.

40. **Thameur H, Chenik S, Abdelmoulah S, Bey M.** *Les localisations Thoraciques de l'hydatidose: à partir de 1619 observations.* Revue de Pneumologie Clinique, 2000, n°56, 1-15.

41. **Kardaras F, Kardara D, Tselikos D, Tsoukas A, Exadactylos N, Anagnostopoulou M et al.** *Fifteen year surveillance of echinococcal heart disease from a referral hospital in Greece.* European heart journal 1996 : 17 ; 1265-70.

42. **Msaad S, Fouzi S, Ayedi H, Ayoub A.** *Pulmonary embolism of hydatid origin: A propos d'un cas.* Rev Tun Infectiol 2009: 3; 29-32.

43. A, Cheniti. *Short- and long-term results of surgical treatment of cardiopericardial hydatid cysts: A propos de 19 observations.* Doctor of Medicine thesis - Sousse 2000.

44. Karadede A, Alyan O, Sucu M, Karahan Z. *Coronary narrowing secondary to compression* by pericardial hydatid cyst. International Journal of Cardiology, 2008, n°123, 204-207.

45. Aissaoui A, Hadj Salem N, Chadly A. *Sudden death due to cardiac hydatidosis.* Journal de médecine légale droit médical 2010 : 53 ; 4.

46. Sinha P.R, Jaipuria N, Avasthey P. *Intracardiac hydatid cyst and sudden death in a child.* International journal of cardiology 1995: 51; 293-5.

47. Ben Hamada K, Maajouk F, Ben Farhaj M. *Eighteen year experience with echinococcosis of the heart: Clinical and echocardiographic features in 14 patients.* International Journal of Cardiology, 2003, 91, 145-151.

48. Rekik S, Krichene S, Sahnoun M, Trabelsi I, Kammoun S. *Unusual cause of syncope in a 17 year-old young woman: Left ventricular hydatid cyst.* International Journal of Cardiology, April, 2008, 77, 12-14.

49. Jaafari A, Boukhriss B et al. *Fatal hydatid pulmonary embolism: A propos de deux observations.* Annales de cardiologie et d'angéiologie 2009: 58; 125-8.

50. Lahdhili H, Hachicha S, Ziadi M, Thameur H. *Acute pulmonary embolism due to the rupture of a right ventricle hydatid cyst.* European journal of cardiothoracic surgery: 2002: 22; 462-4.

51. Beyrouti M.I, Beyrouti R, Abbes I, Khanat M, Ben Ammar M, Frikha F et al. *Acute rupture of hydatid cyst in the peritoneum: A propos de 17 observations.* La presse médicale 2004: 33; 378-384.

52. Kantarci M, Onbas O, Alper F, Celebi Y, Yigiter M, Okur A:. *Anaphylaxis due to a rupture of hydatid cyst: Imaging findings of a 10-year-old boy.* Emergency Radiology 2003: 10: 49-50.

53. Kolsi M, Frikha I, Triki N, Siala I, Ayoub A, Sahnoun Y. *Cardiac localization of multifocal hydatidosis: about a case.* Archive des Maladies du Cœur, 2005, n°98, 75-77.

54. EL Kouby A, Vaillant A, Gomet B. *L'Hydatidose Cardiaque: à propos de 15 cas.* Annales de Cardiologie et d'angéiologie, 1990, n°44, 603-610.

55. Hassine E, Kraoua S, Marniche K, Bousnina S, Lefi A. *Dead and calcified hydatid cyst of the right ventricle: limitation of imaging.* Presse Médicale, 2003, n°32, 1802-4.

56. Porte J, Touboul P, Delahaye JP, Cavallaro J, Clermont A. *Recurrent ventricular tachycardia due to hydatic cyst of the heart.* Archive des Maladies du Cœur et des Vaisseaux, 1975, 68, 893-898.

57. Fertin M, Mouquet F, Lallemant R, Gaxotte V. *Diagnosis Imaging and treatment of unusual cardiac hydatid cyst.* Cardiovascular Pathology, 2006, 15, 356-358.

58. Oueslati S, Saïd W, Saaidi I, Djebbi M, Charrada L, Rezgui L, Menif N, Châabane M. *Imaging of hydatid cyst of the heart: About 8 observations.* Presse Med. 2006; 35: 1162-6.

59. Fortia E, Bendaoud M, Maghur H. *Intracavity cardiac hydatid cyst and the wall sing criteria.* European Journal Ultrasound, 1998, 8, 115-117.

60. Rouetbi N, Saad R, Maatallah A, Mzoughi R. *L'Hypertension Artérielle Pulmonaire post hydatique : à propos d'une observation.* Revues des Maladies Respiratoires, January 2006, 23, 44-45.

61. Ceviz M, Becit N, Kocak H. *Infected Cardiac Hydatid cyst.* Heart, 2001, 86, e13.

62. Sinci V, Ozdogan M.E, Tunaoglu FS, Kula S. *Hydatid disease and massive cardiac involvement.* Annals of Thoracic and Cardiovascular Surgery, Oct, 1999, n°5, 336-339.

63. Hakan M, et al. *Cardiac Hydatid Cyst Located in the Interventricular Septum.* Annals Thorac Surgery, 2002, 74, 21-24.

64. Mrad Dali K, Tlili K, Ly M, Romdhani N, Bakir D, Gharbi H et al. *Radioclinical profile of cardiopericardial hydatid cyst: about 17 cases.* Ann Cardiol Angéiol. 2000; 49: 414-22.

65. Jouhadi Z, Ailal F, Dreoua N, et al. *Cardiac hydatid cyst. Two observations in children.* Presse Med 2004; 33: 1260-3.

66. Baque J, Huart V, Pierrot JM. *Hydatid cyst of the interventricular septum of the heart: appearance on multibar CT and MRI.* Journal de Radiologie, 2003, 84, 614-616.

67. Celik T, et al. *Intracavitary left ventricular hydatid cysts.* International Journal of Cardiology, 2006, 111, 155-157.

68. Vanjak D, Moutaoufik M, Leroy O, Beuscart C, Billiau V, Chidiac C et al. *Cardiac hydatidosis: contribution of magnetic resonance imaging: about a case.* Arch Mal Coeur. 1990; 83: 1739-42.

69. Dursun M, Terzibasioglu E, Yilmaz R, et al. *Cardiac hydatid disease: CT and MRI findings.* . AJR Am J Roentgenol Jan 2008; 190 (1):226-32.

70. Bonardi M, Dellabianca C, Della Valle V, Valentini A, Raineri C, Dore R. *Hydatid cyst of the cardiac interventricular septum.* International Journal of Cardiology 158 (2012) 45-46.

71. Oncel D et al. *A Rare Right Atrial Mass: Hydatid Cys.* European Journal of Radiology Extra, 2007, 61, 87-90.

72. Athanassiadi K, Kalavrouziotis G, Loutsidis A, Bellenis I, Exarchos N. *Surgical treatment of echinococcosis by a transthoracic approach: a* *review of 85 cases.* European journal of cardio-thoracic surgery 1998: 14; 134-40.

73. Mohammad Abbasi MD, Horak Poorzand MD, Nahid Zirak MD, Hamid Hosinikhah MD Chest Pain due to Compression. *Effect of Hydatid Cyst on LAD: Rare Presentation of Hydatid Cyst in Heart.* Iranian Heart Journal 2011; 12 (3): 47-50.

74. Bouree P, Lancon A. *Diagnosis of blood hypereosinophilia.* Revue Française des Laboratoires, April, 2000, 321, 67-71.

75. Salehi M, Soleimani A, et al. *Cardiac Echinococcosis with Negative Serologies: A Report of Two Cases.* Heart Lung and Circulation, 2007, 566, 1-3.

76. DA., Vuitton. *Echinococcosis and allergy .* Clin Rev Allergy Immunol 2004; 26: 93-104.

77. Wellinghausen N, Jo¨chle W, Reuter S, Flegel WA, Gru¨nert A, Kern P. *Zinc status in patients with alveolar echinococcosis is related to disease progression.* Parasite Immunol 1999; 21: 237-241.

78. C, Moulinier. *Parasitology and Medical Mycology: Elements of Morphology and Biology.* Editions Médicales Lavoisier, 2003, Chapter 8: Cestodes, 417-418.

79. Brostein J.A, Klotz F. *Cestodes Larvaires, Encyclopédie Médicochirurgicale.* Maladies Infectieuses. Elsevier, 2005, Chapter 2, 59-83.

80. Yuksel M, Kir A, Ercan S, Fevzi B.H, Baaysungur V. *Correlation between sizes and intracystic pressures of hydatid cysts.* European journal of cardio-thoracic surgery 1997: 12; 903-6.

81. Sarkis A, Ashoush R, Alawi A, Haddad A, Jebara V, Checrallah E. *Hydatid cyst of the heart simulating coronary ischemia.* Ann Cardiol Angéiol 2001: 50; 206-10.

82. Chadly A, Krimi S, Mghirbi T. *Cardiac hydatid cyst rupture as cause of death .* Am J of Forsenic medicine and pathology 2004: 25; 262-4.

83. Di Bello R and al. *Intracardiac rupture of hydatid cyst of the heart.* Circulation, 1963, 27, 366-74.

84. Birincioglu C, Bardakci H, Kucuker S. *A Clinical Cardiac and Pericardiac Echinococcosis.* Annals Thoracic Surgery, 1999, 68, 1290-1294.

85. Uysalel A, Yazicioglu L, Aral A, Akalin H. *A Multi-vesicular Cardiac Hydatid Cyst with Hepatic Involvement.* European Journal of Cardio-thoracic Surgery, 1998, 14, 335-337.

86. Erdogmus B, Yazici B, Ackan Y, Ozdere B.A, Korkmaz U, Alcelic A. *Latent fatality due to hydatid cyst rupture after a severe cough episode.* Tohoku J Exp Med 2005: 205; 293-6.

87. **Maghraoui O.** *Embolie pulmonaire hydatique: Aspects cliniques, radiologiques, thérapeutiques et évolutifs .* Thesis for doctorate in medicine-Tunis 2002.

88. **Ertugrul Mavili, Ali Baykan, Sadettin Sezer, Nazmi Narin.** *A rare cause of pulmonary hypertension: cyst hydatid embolism.* International Journal of Cardiology 140, Supplement 1 (2010) S67.

89. **Béji M, Louzir B, El Mekki F, Jouini S, Mahaouachi R, Daghfous J.** *Post-hydatic chronic pulmonary heart disease.* Rev Mal Resp 1997 : 14 ; 129-31.

90. **Lanzoni AM, Barrios V, Moya JL, Epeldegui A, Lelemin D.** *Dynamic left ventricular outflow obstruction caused by cardiac echinococcosis.* American Heart Journal, 1992, 124, 1083-1085.

91. **Malamou-Misti V, Pappa L, Vougiouklakis T, Peschos D, Kazakos N, Grekas G et al.** *Sudden death due to an unrecognized cardiac hydatid cyst.* Journal of forsenic sciences 2002: 47 (5); 1062-4.

92. **Ozdemir M, Diker E, Aydogdu S, Goksel S.** *Complete heart block caused by cardiac echinococcosis and successfully treated with albendazole.* Heart, 1997, 77, 84-85.

93. **Zied Ibn Elhadj, Marouane Boukhris, Ikram Kammoun, Afef Ben Halima, Faouzi Addad, Salem Kachboura.** *Cardiac hydatid cyst revealed by ventricular tachycardia. .* Journal of the Saudi Heart Association Volume 26, Issue 1, January 2014, Pages 47-50.

94. **Sakarya ME, Etlik O, Sakarya N, et al.** *MR findings in cardiac hydatid cyst.* Clin Imaging May-Jun 2002; 26 (3): 170-2.

95. **Jeroen Walpot, M.D. Bharati Shivalkar, M.D., Ph.D, W. Hans Pasteuning, M.D.and Raymond Hokken, M.D,.** *Staphylococcus aureus Infective Endocarditis mimicking a Hydatid Cyst. .* ECHOCARDIOGRAPHY- AUGUST 2010.

96. **Mehmet Fatih, Ozlu MD, Firat MD, Omac Tufekcioglu.** *Left ventricular apical cyst thrombus mimicking a hydatid cyst.* Can J cardiol vol 25 no 7 2009.

97. **Tetik O, Yılık L, Emrecan B, Ozbek C, Gü¨ rbu¨ z A.** *Giant hydatid cyst in the interventricular septum of a pregnant woman.* Tex Heart Inst J. 2002; 29: 333-335.

98. **Struillou L, Rabaud C, Bischoff N, Preiss M, May T.** *Complications of cardiac hydatid cyst.* La Presse Médicale, Sept, 1997, n°25, 1192-1194.

99. **Cornil A, et al.** *Albendazole: useful in the adjuvant treatment of echinococcosis.* Revue Prescrire, 2000, 207, 416-419.

100. **Koubâa M, Lahiani D, Abid L, Mâaloul I, Ben Kahla S, Bradii M, Marrakchi Ch, Hammami B, Mnif Z, Mnif J, Kammoun S, Ben Jemâa M.** *Can albendazole be the only treatment for cardiac echinococcosis with*

multiple organ involvement? . International Journal of Card 2012;161 :58-60.

101. Jougon J, Delcambre F, Velly JF. *Anterior surgical approaches to the thorax.* EMC Techniques chirurgicales Thorax 2004 : 42-210.

102. Filsoufi F, Fuzellier JF, Fabiani JN. *Surgery of acquired mitral valve I lesions.* EMC Techniques chirurgicales Thorax 1998: 42-530.

103. Noirclerc M, Chauvin G, Fuentes P, Giudicelli R, Le Treut P, Perelman M. *Les thoracotomies* . EMC Techniques chirurgicales Thorax 1986: [42-205].

104. Casselman FP, Slycke CV, Dom H, Lambrechts DL, Vermeulen Y, Vanermen H. *Endoscopic mitral valve repair: feasible, reproducible and durable.* J Thorac Surg 2003; 125: 273-82.

105. Alexandre F., Fabiani J.-N. *Extracorporeal circulation* . EMC (Elsevier Masson SAS, Paris) Techniques chirurgicales - Thorax, 2007; 42-513.

106. W. D. Boyd, N. D. Desai, D. F. D. Rizzo, R. J. Novick, F. N. McKenzie, and A. H. Menkis. *"Off-pump surgery decreases postoperative complications and resource utilization in the elderly."* . Annals of Thoracic Surgery, volume 68, pages 1490-1493, 1999.

107. D. Van Dijk, E. Jansen, and R. e. a. Hijman. *"Cognitive outcome after off-pump and on-pump coronary artery bypass graft surgery."* . Journal of the American Medical Association, vol. 287, no. 11, pages 1405-1412, 2002.

108. Birincioglu CL, Tarcan O, Bardakci H, Saritas A, Tasdemir O. *Off-pump technique for the treatment of ventricular myocardial echinococcosis.* Ann Thorac Surg 2003; 75 (4): 1232-7.

109. Chauvaud S. *Surgery of acquired tricuspid valve lesions.* EMC Techniques chirurgicales-Thorax, 2002; 42-540: 8p.

110. Hicham El Malki, Hicham Benyoussef, Jaafar Rhissassi, Chakib Benlafqih, Abderrahmane Bakkali, Rochde Sayah, Mohamed Laaroussi. *Hydatidosis of the pulmonary infundibulum: an exceptional etiology of right ventricular ejection obstruction About two operated cases.* thoracic and cardiovascular surgery- 2014; 18(1).

111. Chauvaud S. *Surgery of acquired mitral valve lesions: generalities.* EMC Techniques Chirurgicales Thorax 2011: 42-530.

112. Atakan Atalay, Orhan Kemal Salih, Suat Gezerb, Ugur Göcena, Hafize Yaliniz, Vecih Keklik and Yasin Güzel. *Simultaneous Heart and Bilateral Lung Hydatid Cyst Operated in a Single Session.* Heart, Lung and Circulation 2013; 22: 682-684.

113. Maazouzi W, Bennis A. *Hydatid cyst of the heart: from imaging to scalping.* Dar Nachr Almaarrifa, 2001, n°1309.

114 Canpolat U, Yorgun H, Sunman H, Aytemir K. *Cardiac hydatid cyst mimicking left ventricular aneurysm and diagnosed by magnetic resonance imaging.* Turk Kardiyol Dern Ars. 2011; 39(1): 47-51.

115. Kammoun S, Frikha I, Fourati K. *Hydatid cyst of the heart located in the interventricular septum.* Canadian Journal of Cardiology 2000, 56, 41-44.

116. Apaydin, A.Z, Oguz, E, Ayik, F, Nalbantgil, S, Ceylan, N. *Hydatid cyst confined to the papillary muscle: A very rare cause of mitral regurgitation.* Texas Heart Institute Journal Volume 36, Issue 6, 2009, Pages 598-600.

117. Pasaoglu I, Dogan R, Pasaoglu E, Tokgozoglu L. *Surgicaltreatment of giant hydatid cyst of the left ventricle and diagnostic value of magnetic resonance imaging.* . CardiovascSurg 1994; 2:114- 6.

118. Sirlak M, Ozcinara E, Tuncay Erena N, Eryılmaza S, Uysalela A, Ennelia D, Ozyurdaa U. *Multiple hydatid cystectomy of the heart necessitating LIMA to LAD anastomosis in a young patient.* Cardiovascular Pathology 18 (2009) 53-56.

119. Achilleas G. Lioulias, MD John N. Kokotsakis, MD Christophoros N. Foroulis, MD Elian T. Skouteli, MD. *Multiple Cardiac Hydatid Cysts Consistency of Echocardiographic and Surgical Findings.*

120 Akar R, Eryilmaz S, Yazicioglu L, Eren NT, Durdu S, et al. *Surgery for cardiac hydatid disease: an Anatolian experience.* Anadolu Kardiyol Derg 3: 238-44.

121. Ottino G, Villani M, De Paulis R, Trucco G, Viara A. *Restoration of atrioventricular conduction after surgical removal of a hydatid cyst of the interventricular septum.* Journal Thorac Cardiovascular Surgery, 1987, 93, 144-147.

122. C. Levent Birincioglu, MD, Hasmet Bardakci, MD, Seref A. Kucuker. *A Clinical Dilemma: Cardiac and Pericardiac Echinococcosis* . Ann Thorac Surg 1999; 68:1290-4.

123. Eylem Tuncer, Serpil Gezer,Ilkcr Mataraci, Altug Tuncer, Arzu Antal Donmez,Mehmet Aksut, Cevat Yakut. *Surgical Treatment of Cardiac Hydatid Disease in 13 Patients.* Tex Heart Inst J. 2010; 37: 189-193.

124. Murat V, Qian Z, Guo S, Qiao J. *Cardiac and pericardial echinococcosis: report of 15 cases.* Asian Cardiovasc Thorac Ann 15: 278-9.

125. Jerbi S, Kortas C, Dammak S, Hamida N, Aly F, et al. (l. *Cardiopericardial hydatid cyst. Reportof 19 cases.* 2004 Tunis med 82 suppl 1: 152-7.

126. Bouraoui H, Trimeche B, Mahdhaoui A, Majdoub A, Zaaraoui J, et al. *echinococcosis of the heart: clinical and echocardiographic features in 12 patients.* Acta Cardiol 60 :39-41.

127. Kabbani SS, Ramadan A, Kabbani L, Sandouk A, Nabhani F, et al. *surgical experience with caridac echinococcosis.* asian cardiovasc Thoracic ana 15: 422-6.

128. Tasdemir K, Akcali Y, Gunebakmaz O, Kaya MG, Mavili E, et al. *Surgical approach to the management of cardiovascular echinococcosis.* J card Surg 24 : 28.

129. Molavipour A, Javan H, Moghaddam AA, Dastani M, Abbasi M, et al. *Combined medical and surgical treatment of intracardiac hydatid cystsin 11 patients.* J Card Surg 2010 25: 143-6.

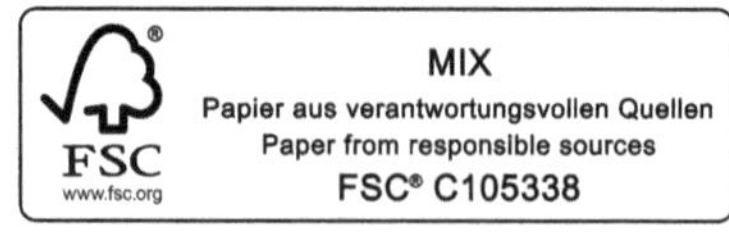

Printed by Books on Demand GmbH, Norderstedt / Germany